The National Collaborating Centre

for Chronic Conditions

Funded to produce guidelines for the NHS by NICE

TYPE 1 DIABETES IN ADULTS

National clinical guideline for diagnosis
and management in primary and secondary care

Published by
ROYAL COLLEGE
OF PHYSICIANS

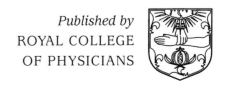

Acknowledgements

The National Collaborating Centre for Chronic Conditions would like to thank Elizabeth Asung, Stora Djumaeva, Jane Ingham, Hilary Jackson, Mike Pearson and Sarah Williams of the National Collaborating Centre for Chronic Conditions for their work and advice on this project, Emma Cox and Bridget Turner of Diabetes UK for their discussion paper on support groups, and Jane Cowl and Victoria Thomas of the Patient Involvement Unit for NICE for their advice and assistance. Thanks are also due to Sue Blakeney, Kevin Shotliffe and Rosemary Walker for attending a meeting as deputies to represent the College of Optometrists, Diabetes UK and the Royal College of Nursing respectively, and Derek Lowe for his expert advice on interpreting statistical aspects of the evidence base. We are also grateful to the National Collaborating Centre for Primary Care for sharing their work on the revised Type 2 diabetes foot care guideline with us.

ROYAL COLLEGE OF PHYSICIANS
11 St Andrews Place, London NW1 4LE

www.rcplondon.ac.uk

Registered charity No 210508

Copyright © 2004 Royal College of Physicians of London
ISBN 1 86016 228 2

Typeset by Dan-Set Graphics, Telford, Shropshire

Printed in Great Britain by Sarum ColourView Group, Salisbury, Wiltshire

Membership of development groups

Consensus Reference Group (CRG)

The names with an asterisk (*) against them were also members of the Guideline Development Group (GDG).

Dr John Astbury, representing the Faculty of Public Health Medicine
Consultant in Health Protection, Health Protection Agency, Cumbria and Lancashire

Ms Clare Bailey, representing the Royal College of Ophthalmologists
Consultant Ophthalmologist, Bristol Eye Hospital

Mr Steven Barnes*
Health Services Research Fellow, National Collaborating Centre for Chronic Conditions

Mr Richard Broughton, representing the College of Optometrists
Community Optometrist, Surrey

Dr Vincent Connelly, representing the Royal College of Physicians of London*
Consultant Physician and Clinical Director, The James Cook University Hospital, Middlesbrough

Dr Melanie Davies, representing Diabetes UK
Consultant Physician in Diabetes and Endocrinology, University Hospitals of Leicester NHS Trust

Mr Richard Edlin*
Research Associate in Health Economics, Sheffield Health Economics Group, University of Sheffield, and Health Economist, National Collaborating Centre for Chronic Conditions

Dr Gary Frost, representing the British Dietetic Association*
Head of Therapy Services and Nutrition & Dietetic Research Group, Imperial College and Hammersmith Hospitals NHS Trust

Dr Roger Gadsby, representing the Royal College of General Practitioners*
GP in Nuneaton, Warwickshire, Senior Lecturer in Primary Care at the University of Warwick and Medical Adviser, Warwick Diabetes Care

Dr Marilyn Gallichan, representing the Royal College of Nursing
Diabetes Specialist Nurse, Royal Cornwall Hospitals Trust

Mr Rob Grant*
Project Manager, National Collaborating Centre for Chronic Conditions

Ms Irene Gummerson, Royal Pharmaceutical Society of Great Britain
Pharmacist, Yorkshire

Ms Debbie Hammond, patient and carer representative representing Diabetes UK*

Dr Simon Heller, Diabetes UK*
Reader in Medicine, University of Sheffield and Honorary Consultant Physician, Sheffield Teaching Hospitals NHS Trust

Professor Philip Home*
Professor of Diabetes Medicine, University of Newcastle upon Tyne, and Clinical Advisor, National Collaborating Centre for Chronic Conditions

Professor Des Johnston
Professor of Endocrinology and Metabolic Medicine, Imperial College and Hammersmith Hospitals NHS Trust, and CRG Chair, National Collaborating Centre for Chronic Conditions

Dr Colin Johnston, representing Diabetes UK
Consultant Physician and Endocrinologist, West Hertfordshire Hospitals NHS Trust

Dr George Kassianos, representing the Royal College of General Practitioners
General Practitioner, Berkshire

Dr Eric Kilpatrick, Association of Clinical Biochemists
Consultant in Chemical Pathology, Hull Royal Infirmary

Ms Suzanne Lucas, patient and carer representative, representing Diabetes UK*

Ms Emma Marcus, representing the British Dietetic Association
Clinical Specialist Diabetes Dietitian, Heart of Birmingham Teaching Primary Care Trust

Dr Alastair Mason*
GDG Lead, National Collaborating Centre for Chronic Conditions

Dr Greg McAnulty, representing the Royal College of Anaesthetists
Consultant in ITU and Anaesthesia, St George's Healthcare NHS Trust

Dr Colin McIntosh, representing Diabetes UK*
Consultant Physician in Diabetes and Endocrinology, Chelsea and Westminster Hospital NHS Trust and Honorary Senior Lecturer, Imperial College London

Ms Sarah O'Brien, Royal College of Nursing*
Nurse Consultant, St Helens and Knowsley Hospitals NHS Trust

Dr Vinod Patel, representing Diabetes UK
Consultant Diabetologist, George Eliot Hospital NHS Trust and Reader in Clinical Skills, University of Warwick Medical School

Ms Karen Reid*
Information Scientist, National Collaborating Centre for Chronic Conditions

Professor Ken Shaw, Royal College of General Practitioners
Consultant Physician and Director of Research & Development, Portsmouth Hospitals NHS Trust, and Association of British Clinical Diabetologists

Mr David Turner, patient and carer representative, representing Diabetes UK*

Ms Barbara Wall, Society of Chiropodists and Podiatrists
Senior Lecturer and Programme Leader for Podiatry, University of East London

The National Collaborating Centre for Women and Children's Health convened a separate guideline development group to develop the children and adolescents' Type 1 diabetes guideline. Dr Vincent Connelly was a member of both groups, helped co-ordinate the work of the two national collaborating centres throughout the process, and chaired the joint meeting of the two GDGs.

Contents

Preface

It is a pleasure to introduce this national guideline on Type 1 diabetes in adults, commissioned by the National Institute for Clinical Excellence (NICE) to identify best practice for the NHS in the management of Type 1 diabetes. It is the fourth such guideline to be prepared by the National Collaborating Centre for Chronic Conditions (NCC-CC) based at the Royal College of Physicians of London.

Type 1 diabetes can, if poorly controlled, produce devastating problems in both the short and the long term. Good control of blood glucose levels reduces the risk of these problems arising, but can be very difficult for patients and carers to achieve. This guideline emphasises that the NHS should provide all patients with the means – and the necessary understanding – to control their diabetes, and that it should help patients integrate the disease management with their other activities and goals. It argues that every person with diabetes should be able to develop their own care plan and utilise effective treatment in a way agreeable to them. The input of various health professionals may be needed to achieve this, and should be readily available. A system of regular monitoring, so that any complications which do develop are picked up at an early stage and treated appropriately, should also be provided.

In common with all NICE guideline recommendations, those for Type 1 diabetes have been developed using a rigorous, evidence-based methodology. An extensive search identified the relevant medical literature, and papers were carefully assessed to ensure that recommendations were based on treatment and practice of proven benefit. This process was carried out by a guideline development group (GDG), a small team from the NCC-CC working together with patients and health professionals with wide expertise in Type 1 diabetes. They have used the available evidence to produce guidance that is clinically relevant as well as methodologically sound. The availability of clinical expertise also allowed recommendations to be made in areas for which there is inadequate evidence, but which are important to patients and carers. At the same time the need for further research in these areas was indentified.

It goes without saying that the members of the GDG deserve enormous thanks for their efforts. The technical team at the NCC-CC, the GDG Lead, the Clinical Advisor and the rest of the group have all worked incredibly hard over the past two years, and have been most generous with their time. Thanks are also due to all those who commented on the guideline at various stages of development. Since I have assumed the directorship of the NCC-CC only at the very end of this process, I can say without any self-aggrandisement that they have done a magnificent job. This full guideline is both an excellent clinical reference work and a practical working document which will improve the care of those with Type 1 diabetes.

Bernard Higgins MD FRCP
Director, National Collaborating Centre for Chronic Conditions

Glossary

ACE inhibitor	Angiotensin-converting enzyme inhibitor.
ADA	American Diabetes Association.
AER	Albumin excretion rate; a measure of kidney damage due to diabetes (and other conditions) and a risk factor for arterial disease.
Albuminuria	The presence of albumin and other proteins in urine.
Alpha-glucosidase inhibitors	Group of drugs which inhibit the digestion of complex carbohydrates in the gut, and thus flatten the post-meal blood glucose excursion.
AMIDA	Active meal-time insulin dose adjustment (see DAFNE).
Autoimmune disease	Condition in which a persons own tissues become the target of attack by their immune system.
Basal-bolus insulin regimen	A meal-time + basal insulin regimen, in which short- or rapid-acting insulin is given before meals, and an extended-acting insulin to cover requirements at night and sometimes between meals.
BGAT	Blood glucose awareness training.
BMI	Body mass index; an index of body weight corrected for height.
CDA	Canadian Diabetes Association.
CGMS	Continuous glucose monitoring systems.
CMAP	Compound muscle action potential.
Cochrane review	The Cochrane Library consists of a regularly updated collection of evidence-based medicine databases including the Cochrane Database of Systematic Reviews (reviews of randomised controlled trials prepared by the Cochrane Collaboration).
Concordance	Concordance is a concept reflecting the extent to which a course of action agreed between clinicians and a person with diabetes is actually carried out; often but not solely used in the sense of therapeutic interventions or behavioural changes.
COPD	Chronic obstructive pulmonary disease.
Cost-effectiveness	Comparative analysis of the costs and health benefits of the treatment or care. In cost effectiveness analysis, the outcomes of different interventions are converted into health gains for which a cost can be associated, for example, cost per diabetic complication prevented.
C-peptide	Biologically inactive part of proinsulin molecule, secreted in equal molar quantities with insulin. C-peptide level gives information on endogenous insulin secretion.
CRG	Consensus Reference Group.
CSII	Continuous subcutaneous insulin infusion; insulin therapy delivered by a pump rather than injection.
DAFNE	Dose adjustment for normal eating; a recent adaptation of a system of self-adjustment of meal-time insulin dose requirement based on assessment of intended food intake.
DCCT	Diabetes Control and Complications Trial; a landmark study of the effects of intensification of diabetes care on development of microvascular complications.
Deep subcutaneous fat	Layer of subcutaneous fat into which insulin has to be injected for optimal effect.
Diabetes centre	A generic term for a source of a unified multidisciplinary diabetes service.

Diabetes mellitus	Chronic condition characterised by elevated blood glucose levels. Diabetes is of diverse aetiology and pathogenesis, and should not be regarded as a single disease. Predominant types are Type 1 diabetes and Type 2 diabetes, diabetes secondary to other pancreatic disease or other endocrine disease, and diabetes of onset in pregnancy.
Diabetes register	A database, at practice, clinic or regional level, including all people diagnosed with diabetes, and containing information on outcomes, complication recall and surveillance, and treatments.
Diabetes UK	Self-help charity for people with diabetes in the UK, and a professional organisation for diabetes care.
DKA	Diabetic ketoacidosis.
DSME	Diabetes self-management education.
ECG	Electrocardiogram.
Education	In the context of this guideline, patient education in self-management of everyday diabetes issues like insulin therapy, dietary changes, self-monitoring of glucose level, physical exercise, foot care, coping with concurrent illness, how to avoid hypoglycaemia, complications, arterial risk control, jobs and travel.
ELISA	Enzyme-linked immunosorbent assay.
EmAb	Anti-endomysial antibodies.
FBG	Fasting blood glucose level or concentration.
Framingham equation	A widely known and used calculation of arterial risk, derived from a long-term study in Framingham, Massachusetts. Not valid in people with Type 1 or Type 2 diabetes.
Fuzzy logic	A logical computing technique, here as used to control insulin infusion on the basis of degrees of certainty of measurements.
GA	Anti-gliadin antibodies; used in the detection of coeliac disease.
GDG	Guideline Development Group.
GFR	Glomerular filtration rate; a measure of kidney function.
GHb	Glycated haemoglobin, see HbA_{1c}.
Glucose excursions	Change in blood glucose levels especially after meals.
Grade (of recommendation)	A code (eg A, B, C) linked to a guideline recommendation, indicating the strength of the evidence supporting that recommendation. The grading does not indicate the importance of the recommendation, nor the certainty of it being true.
HbA_{1c}	The predominant form of glycated haemoglobin, present in red blood cells, and formed when the normal haemoglobin A reacts non-enzymatically with glucose. As the reaction is slow and only concentration dependent, the amount of HbA_{1c} formed is proportional only to the concentration of HbA and glucose. As HbA remains in the circulation for around three months, the amount of HbA_{1c} present, expressed as a percentage of HbA, is proportional to the glucose concentration over that time.
HPLC	High performance liquid chromatography; one method used in the measurement of HbA_{1c}.
HTA	Health technology assessment; funded by the NHS Research and Development Directorate.
ICA	Islet cell antibodies (see islet B cells).
IDF	International Diabetes Federation; a global federation of diabetes associations.
IgA	Immunoglobulin A.
IGT	Impaired glucose tolerance; a condition of hyperglycaemia less marked by diabetes but association with a high risk of arterial damage.

Insulin analogues	A derivative of human insulin in which change of the amino-acid sequence alters duration of action after injection.
Insulin regimen	A therapeutic combination of different insulin preparations, including time of injection and frequency during a day.
ISDN	Isosorbide dinitrate.
Islet B-cell; sometimes β-cells	Located in the islets of Langerhans of the pancreas, the cells which produce insulin.
Isophane insulin	A synonym for NPH (neutral protamine Hagedorn) insulin.
ISPAD	International Society for Paediatric and Adolescent Diabetes.
Lente insulin	A basal insulin, made by combining insulin with large amounts of zinc; first available in 1951.
MCV	Motor conduction velocity.
MDI	Multiple daily injections (*see* basal-bolus insulin regimen).
Metabolic syndrome	Overweight (abdominal adiposity), insulin insensitivity, higher blood pressure, abnormal blood fat profile.
Methodological limitations	Features of the design or reporting of a clinical study which are known to be associated with risk of bias or lack of validity. Where a study is reported in this guideline as having significant methodological limitations, a recommendation has not been directly derived from it.
Microalbuminuria	A low but clinically significant level of albumin and other proteins in the urine.
MNCV	Motor nerve conduction velocity.
MODY	Maturity onset diabetes in the young, a dominant gene disorder, not to be confused with Type 1 diabetes, and not insulin dependent.
Multidisciplinary team	Team of people of differing expertise; for diabetes care with expertise in patient education, prevention, therapy, management of complications, foot care, diet, counselling and the like.
NCC-CC	The National Collaborating Centre for Chronic Conditions, set up in 2000 to undertake commissions from NICE to develop clinical guidelines for the NHS.
NHS	National Health Service. This guideline is written for the NHS in England and Wales.
NICE	National Institute for Clinical Excellence; a special health authority set up within the NHS to develop appropriate and consistent advice on health care technologies, and to commission evidence-based guidelines.
NPH insulin	Neutral protamine Hagedorn insulin, a basal insulin, named after the Danish researcher Hans Christian Hagedorn, and developed in the 1940s. Synonymous with isophane insulin.
NPT	Near patient testing.
NSC	National Screening Committee (UK).
NSF	National Service Framework; a nationwide initiative designed to improve delivery of care for a related group of conditions.
OGTT	Oral glucose tolerance test; a diagnostic test sometimes used in people with equivocal diabetes.
PDE5 inhibitors	Phosphodiesterase type 5 inhibitors, a class of drugs developed in recent years to treat erectile dysfunction.
PPAR-γ agonists	A group of drugs which improve insulin sensitivity in people with reduced sensitivity to their own or injected insulin; presently the licensed drugs are both of the chemical group known as thiazolidinediones (trivially 'glitazones').

PROCAM	Prospective Cardiovascular Münster Heart Study – an epidemiological study performed in Germany.
Proteinuria	The presence of protein in the urine.
QALY	Quality-adjusted life year; a measure of a person's quality of life, used here in the sense of loss of quality through disease, and gain in quality through health care interventions.
RCT	Randomised clinical trial; a trial in which people are randomly assigned to two (or more) groups: one (the experimental group) receiving the treatment that is being tested, and the other (the comparison or control group) receiving an alternative treatment, a placebo (dummy treatment) or no treatment. The two groups are followed up to compare differences in outcomes to see how effective the experimental treatment was. Such trial designs help minimise experimental bias.
RDW	Red cell distribution width.
Rigiscan	An instrument used in research to measure penile tumescence and rigidity.
SIGN	Scottish Intercollegiate Guidelines Network.
SNAP	Sensory nerve action potential.
SWM	Semmes-Weinstein monofilament.
Technology appraisal	Formal ascertainment and review of the evidence surrounding a health technology, restricted in the current document to appraisals undertaken by NICE.
Type 1 diabetes	Insulin-deficiency disease, developing predominantly in childhood, characterized by hyperglycaemia if untreated, and with a consequent high risk of vascular damage using developing over a period of decades.
Type 2 diabetes	Diabetes generally of slow onset mainly found in adults and in association with features of the metabolic syndrome. Carries a very high risk of vascular disease. While not insulin-dependent, many people with the condition eventually require insulin therapy for optimal blood glucose control.
UKDIABS	A large study/initiative of the collection of outcomes and process data from diabetes care services throughout the UK.
UKPDS	United Kingdom Prospective Diabetes Study – a landmark study of the effect of different diabetes therapies on vascular complications in people with Type 2 diabetes.
VO$_2$max	The oxygen consumption of a person exercising maximally.
VPT	Vibratory perception threshold.
WHO	World Health Organization.

THE DEVELOPMENT OF THE GUIDELINE

1 | Introduction

The word 'diabetes' refers to a group of disorders with a number of common features, of which raised blood glucose is the most evident. In England and Wales the three most common types of diabetes are:

- Type 1 diabetes
- Type 2 diabetes
- gestational diabetes (diabetes of pregnancy).

This guideline is concerned only with Type 1 diabetes. The underlying disorder is that of a pure hormone deficiency disease: lack of insulin. Because hormone replacement with insulin therapy is suboptimal, and despite the implementation of lifestyle and disease management measures, acute and long-term complications are endemic.

In people whose diabetes is untreated, glucose metabolism may be sufficiently disturbed to cause symptoms, typically of polyuria, thirst, weight loss and fatigue. With further worsening, diabetic coma (ketoacidosis) may occur due to disturbed fat metabolism.

Because insulin therapy, problematically, can give rise to high and low blood glucose levels, people with diabetes have to engage in a high level of self-care to contain the risk of acute and late complications.

The main complications of diabetes in the longer term are:

- eye, kidney, and nerve damage
- arterial disease affecting the heart, brain and feet.

In many people with Type 1 diabetes, abnormalities of blood pressure and blood lipids also develop, particularly in association with diabetic kidney damage. In such people there is a very high risk of premature arterial disease.

1.1   Definition

The Guideline Development Group (GDG, see 2.2) worked to the World Health Organization (WHO) definition of Type 1 diabetes,

> a condition of deficiency of insulin secretion from the pancreas, usually due to auto-immune damage of the insulin producing cells. However the clinical condition is generally recognised on the basis of diabetes (high blood glucose levels) occurring in mainly younger and thinner people in the absence of other precipitating causes.[8]

The GDG were, however, conscious that some people with evident Type 1 diabetes and thus absolute insulin deficiency, also have insulin insensitivity in the context of the metabolic syndrome (overweight, insulin insensitivity, higher blood pressure, abnormal blood fat profile).

It was noted that Type 2 diabetes in the young, and the condition known as maturity onset diabetes in the young (MODY), should not be confused with Type 1 diabetes. This is mainly an issue of definition of Type 2 diabetes or MODY rather than Type 1 diabetes. Some conditions of pancreatic damage have a similar phenotype to Type 1 diabetes, but these are usually obvious and of little consequence to the management of the diabetes, so are not considered further.

1.2 Health and resource burden

Type 1 diabetes can result in a wide range of complications, and these affect both the individual patient and the National Health Service. The economic impact of the disease includes:

- direct cost to the NHS
- indirect cost to the economy, including the effects of early mortality
- personal impact of diabetes and subsequent complications on patients and their families.

The direct cost of Type 1 diabetes to the NHS was estimated to be £96m in 1992 prices,[1] which corresponds to approximately £167m at 2001 prices and population levels. The GDG adjusted this figure, using more recent data and expert judgement, to correct for the underestimate of some components[2,3] and to reflect changes in standard treatment, and arrived at a figure of £212m in 2001 prices. The figure includes:

- renal replacement therapy costs of £38m
- outpatient support costs of £50m
- hospitalisation costs of £65m.

Whilst the indirect costs of diabetes are difficult to quantify, in 1992 the costs in terms of lost productivity were estimated to be slightly higher than the direct costs of Type 1 diabetes.[1]

1.3 Scope

The recommendations in the guideline are subject to a number of limitations. The sponsoring authority, NICE, is primarily concerned with health services in England and Wales, so the guideline only indirectly refers to:

- social services
- the voluntary sector
- employers
- services supplied by secondary and tertiary specialties for the late complications of diabetes (for example renal, cardiological, urological and opthalmological services)
- the education sector (including schools and universities)
- others concerned with an individual's health, rather than healthcare.

Nonetheless, the importance of other agencies must not be ignored, and in each locality the aim should be to integrate care for people with Type 1 diabetes across all relevant sectors.

A pre-agreed scope (see Appendix C) defined the remit of the guideline and specified which aspects of Type 1 diabetes would be included and excluded. The scope had been through stakeholder consultation in accordance with processes established by NICE[4] before the development of the guideline began, and covered both a children's guideline and this guideline for adults. It specified that the groups to be covered were to include babies, children, adolescents, adults, and older people with Type 1 diabetes.

Because NICE is considering developing a separate guideline on diabetes in pregnancy, the scope did not cover:

- the management of women with diabetes who wish to conceive or who are pregnant
- the management of women who develop diabetes during pregnancy.

The guideline scope covered the following health settings:

- care received from primary and secondary healthcare professionals who have direct contact with and advise on the care of people with Type 1 diabetes
- the interface between community and specialist care, including the circumstances in which people should be referred or admitted to specialist care both within diabetes care and to other specialties
- the interface between children's and adult services
- support/advice that the NHS should offer to crèches, nurseries, schools and other institutions.

The scope also details the aspects of clinical management to be addressed (see Appendix C).

1.4 Other relevant work

This guideline has been developed with the knowledge that other national work on diabetes has been completed or is in progress. Work on diabetes not commissioned by NICE includes:

- the National Service Framework for diabetes, developed by the Department of Health (**www.dh.gov.uk**)
- an information strategy, developed by the NHS Information Authority (**www.nhsia.nhs.uk/phsmi/datasets/pages/diabetes.asp**)
- guidance on health outcome indicators, developed by the National Centre for Health Outcomes Development[5]
- a system of national clinical audit, set up by the Commission for Health Improvement (**www.nhsia.nhs.uk/ncasp/pages/default.asp**)
- a report for HM Treasury which aims to provide an evidence-based assessment of long-term resource requirements for the NHS, and includes information on diabetes (Chapter 6). *Securing our future health: taking a long-term view*, also known as the First Wanless Report, is available from (**www.hm-treasury.gov.uk/ consultations_and_legislation/wanless/consult_wanless_final.cfm**)

NICE has commissioned these other guidelines on diabetes:

- Type 2 diabetes (completed):
  - guideline E, retinopathy
  - guideline F, renal disease prevention and early management
  - guideline G, blood glucose management and patient education
  - guideline H, blood pressure and blood lipid management
  - guideline 10, foot care (updated).

NICE has commissioned the following technical appraisals relevant to diabetes:

- Type 1 and Type 2 diabetes (completed):
  - appraisal 53, long-acting insulin analogues
  - appraisal 57, insulin pump therapy
  - appraisal 60, patient education models

- Type 2 diabetes (completed):
  - appraisal 9, rosiglitazone
  - appraisal 21, proglitazone
  - appraisal 63, glitazones
- Type 1 and Type 2 diabetes (completed):
  - appraisal 71, coronary artery stents
  - appraisal 73, myocardial perfusion scintigraphy
- Type 1 and Type 2 diabetes (in development):
  - coronary events: statins.

2 | Methodology

2.1　Aims and principles

This chapter describes the resources and techniques used to reach the clinical recommendations in this guideline.

Clinical guidelines have been formally defined as 'systematically developed statements to assist both practitioner and patient decisions in specific circumstances'.[6] This guideline aims to offer the best practice advice on the care of adults (defined as those aged 18 years or older) with Type 1 diabetes. It gives guidance on the management, monitoring and support of people with Type 1 diabetes. The context of the intended guidance is the primacy of the needs of the individual with diabetes, reflecting the difficulties of reconciling the problems of insulin replacement therapy with personal lifestyles.

The current guideline is aimed at helping all healthcare professionals provide optimal services for people with Type 1 diabetes by:
- providing healthcare professionals with a set of explicit statements on the best known ways to assist people with diabetes with their most common clinical problems, while maximising the effectiveness of the service in supporting the population with Type 1 diabetes
- giving commissioning organisations and provider services specific guidance on the best way to provide complex services in a way that maximises efficiency and equity (service organisation is, however, outside the scope of this clinical guideline)
- informing people with diabetes of the optimal methods for helping them self-manage their diabetes.

Others, including the general public, may find the guideline of use in understanding the global and clinical approach to Type 1 diabetes. Separate short-form documents for the public and for healthcare professionals are available; they summarise the recommendations without giving full details of the supporting evidence.

The main principles behind the development of this guideline are that it should:
- consider all the most important issues in the management of people with Type 1 diabetes using published evidence wherever this is available
- be useful to and usable by all professionals
- take full account of the perspectives of the person with Type 1 diabetes and their carers
- indicate areas of uncertainty or controversy needing further research.

2.2　The developers

▷　The National Collaborating Centre for Chronic Conditions

The National Collaborating Centre for Chronic Conditions (NCC-CC) is housed by the Royal College of Physicians (RCP) but governed by a multiprofessional partners board, which includes patient groups and NHS management. It was set up in 2000 to undertake commissions from the National Institute for Clinical Excellence (NICE) to develop clinical guidelines for the NHS in England and Wales.

▷ The technical team

The technical team consisted of:

- an information scientist
- a health services research fellow
- a clinical advisor
- a health economist
- the chair of the Guideline Development Group (GDG)
- a project manager

and was supported by administrative personnel. It took part in the GDG meetings, and also met separately each month.

▷ The Guideline Development Group

The GDG met monthly for 10 months to review the evidence identified by the technical team, to comment on its completeness and to develop and refine clinical recommendations based on that evidence and other considerations.

Editorial responsibility for this guideline rests solely with the GDG.

Nominations for group members were invited from various stakeholder organisations, which were selected to ensure an appropriate mix of clinical professions and patient groups. These made up the Consensus Reference Group (CRG, see below) and from their members the GDG was selected to represent the groups involved in the day-to-day management of Type 1 diabetes. It included two representatives of people with Type 1 diabetes. Each nominee was expected to serve as an individual expert in their own right and not as a mandated representative, although they were encouraged to keep their parent organisation informed of the process. Group membership details can be found at the front of this document.

All group members made a formal 'declaration of interests' at the start of the guideline development and provided updates throughout. The NCC-CC and the GDG Chair monitored these.

▷ The Consensus Reference Group

The larger Consensus Reference Group (CRG) met twice during the process, once early in the development to ensure the aims and clinical questions (see Appendix A) were appropriate, and again at the end of the process to review the validity of the recommendations drafted by the GDG. The formal consensus technique used for this purpose was developed by the NCC-CC and is a modification of the RAND Nominal Group Technique.

▷ Involvement of people with Type 1 diabetes

The NCC-CC believes that the views of people with diabetes and their carers are an integral part of the development process of a guideline on Type 1 diabetes. Patient organisation representation (Diabetes UK) was secured on the Guideline Development Group and included a non-healthcare professional with Type 1 diabetes. People with diabetes were also present as part of the GDG and CRG and were involved at every stage of the guideline development process.

2.3   Searching for the evidence

There were four stages to evidence identification and retrieval:

1   The technical team set out a series of specific clinical questions (see Appendix A) that covered the issues identified in the project scope. The CRG met to discuss, refine and approve these questions as suitable for identifying appropriate evidence from within the published literature.

2   A total of 74 questions were identified. The technical team and project executive agreed that a full literature search and critical appraisal process could not be undertaken for all of these areas due to the time limitations of the guideline development process. The technical team identified questions where it was felt that a full literature search and critical appraisal were essential. Reasons for this included an awareness of new or unclear evidence, or a particular clinical need for evidence-based guidance in the area.

3   The information scientist, with the assistance of the clinical advisor, developed a search strategy for each question to identify the available evidence. Identified titles and abstracts were reviewed for relevance to the agreed clinical questions and full papers obtained as appropriate. These were assessed for inclusion according to predefined criteria as developed by the Scottish Intercollegiate Guidelines Network (SIGN).

4   The full papers were critically appraised by the health services research fellow and the pertinent data entered into evidence tables. These were then reviewed and analysed by the GDG as the basis upon which recommendations were formulated.

Due to the large amount of literature potentially relevant to Type 1 diabetes, the inclusion criteria aimed to limit the included studies to those of a higher level (see 2.6) conducted primarily in people with Type 1 diabetes. Where these were not available, lower-level studies, well-conducted studies outside Type 1 diabetes (in Type 2 diabetes or in the non-diabetic population), or more methodologically-limited studies in people with Type 1 diabetes, were included.

Limited details of the databases and constraints used in the searches can be found in Appendix A. No formal contact was made with the authors of identified studies. Additional contemporary articles identified by the GDG on an *ad hoc* basis, and further published evidence identified by national stakeholder organisations, were incorporated where appropriate after having been assessed for inclusion by the same criteria as evidence provided by the electronic searches.

Searches were rerun at the end of the guideline development process, thus including evidence published and included in the literature databases up to 27 May 2003. Studies recommended by stakeholders or GDG members that were published after this date were not considered for inclusion. The date should be the starting point for searching for new evidence for future updates to this guideline.

2.4   Synthesising the evidence

Abstracts of articles identified by the searches were screened for relevance, and hard copies were ordered of papers that appeared to provide useful evidence relevant to each clinical question. Using a validated appraisal tool, each paper was assessed for its methodological quality against pre-defined criteria. Papers that met the inclusion criteria were then assigned a level according to the evidence hierarchy given under 2.6. Owing to practical limitations, selection, critical appraisal and data extraction were undertaken by one reviewer only. Evidence was, however, considered carefully by the GDG for accuracy and completeness.

Each clinical question dictated the study design that was prioritised in the search strategy. In addition, certain topics within any one clinical question at times required different evidence types to be considered. Randomised control trials (RCTs) were the most appropriate study design for some clinical questions as they lend themselves particularly well to research into medicines. They were not, however, appropriate for all clinical questions, for example the evaluation of diagnostic tests.

RCTs are difficult to perform in areas such as rehabilitation and lifestyle, where interventions are often tailored to the needs of the individual. As a consequence, pharmaceutical interventions tend to be placed higher in the evidence hierarchy than other, equally important, interventions. This should not be interpreted as a preference for a particular type of intervention or as a reflection of the quality of the evidence, particularly for those clinical areas where non-RCT evidence is valid and most appropriate.

Where available, evidence from well-conducted systematic reviews was appraised and presented. Trials included within these reviews are listed in the evidence table but were not critically appraised. Studies identified in addition to those included in the systematic review were included in the appraisal process.

At times, evidence was not available from studies that included a Type 1 diabetes population. Where a Type 2 or mixed diabetes population, or non-diabetes population, is considered, it is indicated in the relevant evidence statement.

On occasion the group identified a clinical question that could not be appropriately answered through undertaking a rigorous literature review (because the evidence was scarce, or conflicting). These questions were addressed by group consensus, and the group considered a summary of the area in an expert-drafted discussion paper. In these instances there was no formal assessment of the studies cited.

Finally, national and international evidence-based guidelines were referred to during the development process. These were not formally appraised because of the consistency of process and of evidence base can be difficult to ascertain across such documents.

The evidence statements should be read with the following caveats in mind:
- all comparisons discussed are statistically significant unless otherwise stated
- where evidence is available from a good quality systematic review or meta-analysis, then individual studies are not reviewed and referenced. Any additional RCT evidence presented relates to studies published since the completion of systematic review(s) included or those considered relevant to this guideline, but which may not have been suitable for inclusion in the systematic review(s)
- unless explicitly stated, all studies relate to diabetes populations. The inclusion of studies of Type 1, Type 2 or mixed Type 1 and Type 2 diabetes populations varies between questions (see Appendix A)
- descriptions of studies of poor methodological quality in evidence statements include details on all relevant interventions in a specified question. However, no positive recommendations have been based solely on such studies

- evidence statements in this guideline derived from one systematic review may be graded with different hierarchy of evidence in different places, due to some topics within the review being based on a synthesis of the outcomes of well-conducted randomised controlled trials and others being based on a synthesis of non-randomised studies, prevalance studies and diagnotic studies, or on consensus
- when other guidelines are reviewed, some of their recommendations are presented here as evidence statements. These may not necessarily reflect the recommendations made in this guideline and are clearly labelled
- where individual trials are referred to in the evidence statements as small, medium, or large, this equates to the following number of participants (at baseline): small, less than 50; medium, from 50 to 200; large, greater than 200. Exact numbers for each trial can be found in the online evidence tables.

2.5   Health economic evidence

While evidence on cost-effectiveness was extracted from the clinical literature searches wherever it existed, this was rare. As such, a separate search was conducted to isolate the health economic evidence that attempted to identify the cost of, and the benefits accruing from, each strategy or intervention. An *a priori* study design criterion was not imposed, so information may come from sources other than RCTs and formal economic evaluations.

As the management of diabetes is complex, many of the areas covered by this guideline have little economic evidence; within clinical trials it is not always clear which of a range of interventions and strategies actually improves health. The GDG therefore expected the useful cost-effectiveness evidence to fall within a limited range of areas. Where searching produced either no evidence or insufficient evidence for a substantive health economic evidence statement, this fact is indicated.

The health economist presented the economic evidence to the GDG alongside the clinical evidence. There is no standard measure to assess the quality of the economic evidence, and reported costs and benefits experienced in other healthcare systems may not apply in the UK. The GDG had to assess not only the results but also their applicability.

Health economic analysis can provide a framework for combining information from a variety of sources to form a standard comparison of cost and benefits. However, the task of producing these estimates is complex and labour intensive, and requires a level of clinical evidence that is not always readily available. Evidence on the costs and benefits of a broad range of interventions was presented to the GDG, but the issue of cultured human dermis for foot ulceration was identified as a particularly important area for further economic analysis. The choice was made on the grounds that:

- this treatment does not have good quality economic evidence attached
- it has a potentially large health benefit
- if made available, the treatment could have a large effect on NHS resources given the prevalence of diabetic foot ulcers
- there are uncertainties surrounding both the benefits and resources, and an absence of cost-utility studies.

2.6   Drafting recommendations

Evidence for each topic was extracted into tables and summarised in evidence statements. The GDG reviewed the evidence tables and statements at each meeting and reached a group opinion. Recommendations were explicitly linked to the evidence supporting them and graded according to the level of the evidence upon which they were based, using the grading system in the table below.

It should be noted that it is the level of evidence that determines the grade assigned to each recommendation. The grade does not necessarily reflect the clinical importance attached to the recommendation.

Hierarchy of evidence		Typical grading of recommendations	
Ia	Evidence from meta-analysis of randomised controlled trials.	A	Based on category I evidence.
Ib	Evidence from at least one randomised controlled trial.		
IIa	Evidence from at least one controlled study without randomisation.	B	Based on category II evidence or extrapolated from category I.
IIb	Evidence from at least one other type of quasi-experimental study.		
III	Evidence from non-experimental descriptive studies, such as comparative studies, correlation studies and case control studies.	C	Based on category III evidence or extrapolated from category I or II.
IV	Evidence from expert committee reports or opinions and/or clinical experience of respected authorities.	D	Directly based on category IV evidence or extrapolated from category I, II or III.
DS	Evidence from diagnostic studies.	DS	Evidence from diagnostic studies.
NICE	Evidence from NICE guidelines or health technology appraisal programme.	NICE	Evidence from NICE guidelines or health technology appraisal programme.

2.7   Agreeing recommendations

Once the evidence review had been completed and an early draft of the guideline produced, a one-day meeting of the CRG was held to finalise the recommendations. This included a pre-meeting vote on the recommendations and a further vote at the CRG meeting, where the group was asked to consider the draft guideline in two stages:

1   Are the evidence-based statements acceptable and is the evidence cited sufficient to justify the grading attached?

2   Are the recommendations derived from the evidence justified and are they sufficiently practical so that those at the clinical front line can implement them? Three types of recommendation were considered:

   a)   A recommendation from the GDG based on strong evidence, usually non-controversial unless there was important evidence that had been missed or misinterpreted

b) A recommendation that was based on good evidence but where it was necessary to extrapolate the findings to make it useful in the NHS. The extrapolation was approved by consensus

c) Recommendations for which no evidence existed but which address important aspects of care, and for which a consensus on best practice could be reached.

This formal consensus method has been established within the NCC-CC, drawing on the knowledge set out in a health technology appraisal,[7] the work of the Royal College of Nursing Institute[1] and practical experience. It approximates to a modification of the RAND Nominal Group Technique and will be fully described in future publications.

2.8 Writing the guideline

The draft version of the guideline was drawn up by the technical team in accordance with the decisions of the guideline groups. Prior to publication, it was circulated to stakeholders according to the formal NICE stakeholder consultation and validation phase.

Modifications were made to this document in response to comments received. Changes were approved by the Guideline Development Group, who retain the final editorial authority for the content.

2.9 Structure of the guideline

The part of this document which contains recommendations (chapter 4 onwards) is divided into sections, each of which covers a set of related topics. For each topic the layout is the same:

- the **rationale** for including the topic is provided in one or two paragraphs that simply set the recommendations in the context of their clinical importance
- the **evidence statements**, both clinical and health economic, are then given, summarising the evidence (more detail can be found in the **evidence tables**, available on the web at **www.rcplondon.ac.uk/pubs/books/dia/index.asp**) Specific health economic evidence statements also follow the clinical evidence when available. The evidence statements and tables aim to contextualise and explain each recommendation
- the evidence statements are followed by a **consideration** that reflects the thinking of the GDG in making the recommendations. This is intended to explain how the evidence was used to formulate the recommendations
- the **recommendations** follow. These are graded to indicate the level of the evidence behind the recommendation, rather than how valid the GDG believes them to be. In some sections of the guideline, additional text providing more detailed guidance is contained within the recommendations.

3 | Key messages of the guideline

3.1 Key recommendations

Patient-centred care

1 The views and preferences of individuals with Type 1 diabetes should be integrated into their healthcare. Diabetes services should be organised, and staff trained, to allow and encourage this.

Multidisciplinary team approach

2 The range of professional skills needed for delivery of optimal advice to adults with diabetes should be provided by a multidisciplinary team. Such a team should include members having specific training and interest to cover the following areas of care:
- education/information giving
- nutrition
- therapeutics
- identification and management of complications
- foot care
- counselling
- psychological care.

Patient education

3 Culturally appropriate education should be offered after diagnosis to all adults with Type 1 diabetes (and to those with significant input into the diabetes care of others). It should be repeated as requested and according to annual review of need. This should encompass the necessary understanding, motivation and skills to manage appropriately:
- blood glucose control (insulin, self-monitoring, nutrition)
- arterial risk factors (blood lipids, blood pressure, smoking)
- late complications (feet, kidney, eye, heart).

Blood glucose control

4 Blood glucose control should be optimised towards attaining DCCT-harmonised HbA_{1c} targets for prevention of microvascular disease (7.5% or lower) and, in those at increased risk, arterial disease (6.5% or lower) as appropriate, while taking into account:
- the experiences and preferences of the insulin user, in order to avoid hypoglycaemia
- the necessity to seek advice from professionals knowledgeable of the range of available mealtime and basal insulins and of optimal combinations thereof, and their optimal use.

Arterial risk factor control

5 Adults with Type 1 diabetes should be assessed for arterial risk at annual intervals. Those found to be at increased risk should be managed through appropriate interventions and regular review. Note should be taken of:

- microalbuminuria, in particular
- the presence of features of the metabolic syndrome
- conventional risk factors (family history, abnormal lipid profile, raised blood pressure, smoking).

Late complications

6 Adults with Type 1 diabetes should be assessed for early markers and features of eye, kidney, nerve, foot, and arterial damage at annual intervals. According to assessed need, they should be offered appropriate interventions and/or referral in order to reduce the progression of such late complications into adverse health outcomes affecting quality of life.

3.2 An outline Type 1 diabetes care algorithm

Initial review

Annual review

Diagnosis and assessment (and acute care if needed)

Initial education and skill acquisition

Annual assessment of education and skills

Education/skill deficits belief/empowerment problems

Annual assessment of arterial risk factors against targets

Abnormal cardiovascular risk factors

Annual assessment of developing complications

Developing complications

Adjustment of insulin doses and insulin regimen

Assessment of blood glucose control against targets

Structured education, lifestyle and nutrition

Assessment of diabetes education and skills

Cardiovascular risk factor interventions

Assessment of cardiovascular risk factors against targets

Specific interventions or referral

More frequent assessment of developing complications

Regular review

3.3 Audit criteria

The audit criteria shown below are linked to the key messages in 3.1. These are intended to be suggestions to aid and monitor the implementation of this guideline at the level of an NHS trust or similar scale healthcare provider.

Table 1: Audit criteria for key messages

Key message	Audit criterion	Exceptions	Definition
Patient-centred care			
1. The views and preferences of individuals with Type 1 diabetes should be integrated into their healthcare. Diabetes services should be organised, and staff trained, to allow and encourage this.	Method: Structured records should show evidence, for every individual with diabetes, that their agenda and views are being incorporated into agreed clinical decisions. Measure: Percent with such evidence within the previous 12 months.	None.	Structured record fields may show evidence of responses to open questions, the person's views on taking an agreed decision recorded, and/or the person's personal targets noted.
Multidisciplinary team approach			
2. The range of professional skills needed for delivery of optimal advice to adults with diabetes should be provided by a multidisciplinary team. Such a team should include members having specific training and interest to cover the following areas of care: • education/information giving • nutrition • therapeutics • identification and management of complications • foot care • counselling • psychological care.	The diabetes service should include, working together as a team, people with specific and maintained training in medical, educational, dietetic, and foot-care aspects of diabetes care. Method: Record whether each aspect is present. Measure: Percent with such evidence within the previous 12 months.	None.	The professional members of the care 'team' are the people who habitually work together to help individual people with diabetes. 'Training' means formal training where that exists for the healthcare professional type, or otherwise training by suitable experience with expert colleagues. 'Training' implies that continuing professional education is undertaken by all team members.

continued

Table 1: Audit criteria for key messages – continued

Key message	Audit criterion	Exceptions	Definition
Patient education			
3. Culturally appropriate education should be offered after diagnosis to all adults with Type 1 diabetes (and to those with significant input into the diabetes care of others). It should be repeated as requested and according to annual review of need. This should encompass the necessary understanding, motivation, and skills to manage appropriately: ● blood glucose control (insulin, self-monitoring, nutrition) ● arterial risk factors (blood lipids, blood pressure, smoking) ● late complications (feet, kidney, eye, heart).	*Newly diagnosed* Method: The medical notes should record within the six months after diagnosis progress through a culturally-appropriate structured education programme designed for people with Type 1 diabetes and covering lifestyle and medical topics. Measure: Percent of records with such evidence. *Subsequent years* Method: The medical notes should record within the previous 14 months an assessment of agreed and culturally-appropriate educational needs, and delivery of education to meet those needs. Measure: Percent of records with such evidence.	None.	An education programme is a structured activity involving health-care professional trained in the principles of adult education. 'Culturally appropriate' implies that attention is paid to beliefs, education attainment, desires, lifestyle, and language in devising and delivering the programme to the individual.
Blood glucose control			
4. Blood glucose control should be optimised towards attaining DCCT-harmonised HbA_{1c} targets for prevention of microvascular disease (7.5% or lower) and, in those at increased risk, arterial disease (6.5% or lower) as appropriate, while taking into account: ● the experiences and preferences of the insulin user, in order to avoid hypoglycaemia ● the necessity to seek advice from professionals knowledgeable of the range of available mealtime and basal insulins and of optimal combinations thereof, and their optimal use.	*General glucose control* Method: The medical record should note those with Type 1 diabetes diagnosed longer than one year who have HbA_{1c} ≥7.5% measured with a DCCT-harmonised assay, and recorded at last annual review within the previous 14 months or if no annual review at last regular review within 12 months. Measure: Percentage 7.5% or lower, with statistical trend to improvement in recent years or in best quartile when benchmarked against equivalent other services. *Hypoglycaemia* Method: Patient records should note episodes of severe hypoglycaemia. Measure: Percentage experiencing one or more episodes of severe hypoglycaemia within the last 12 months.	People with haemoglobinopathies or abnormalities of erythrocyte turnover.	DCCT-harmonisation means traceability of the assay standardisation to NGSP reference standards (or to the IFCC standard, with adjustment to the DCCT norm), and participation in a national quality assurance scheme.

continued

Table 1: Audit criteria for key messages – continued

Key message	Audit criterion	Exceptions	Definition
Arterial risk factor control			
5. Adults with Type 1 diabetes should be assessed for arterial risk at annual intervals. Those found to be at increased risk should be managed through appropriate interventions and regular review. Note should be taken of: • microalbuminuria, in particular • the presence of features of the metabolic syndrome • conventional risk factors (family history, abnormal lipid profile, raised blood pressure, smoking).	*Assessment* Method: The medical record should give a structured record of assessment of cardiovascular risk factors within the previous 14 months. Measure: Percentage of records with such records. *Subsequent management* Method: The medical record should plan for management where microalbuminuria diagnosed, smoker, LDL cholesterol >2.6 mmol/l, triglycerides >2.3 mmol/l, systolic or diastolic blood pressure >135/85 mmHg, and change in first degree family history of cardiovascular events, or any previous personal cardiovascular event or history. Measure: Percent with such plans.	None.	Non-glucose cardiovascular risk factors include: abnormal albumin excretion rate (albumin/ creatinine ratio or sometimes urinary albumin concentration), smoking, blood pressure, full lipid profile (including HDL and LDL cholesterol and triglycerides), age, family history of cardiovascular disease (CVD) and abdominal adiposity.
Late complications			
6. Adults with Type 1 diabetes should be assessed for early markers and features of eye, kidney, nerve, foot, and arterial damage at annual intervals. According to assessed need, they should be offered appropriate interventions and/or referral in order to reduce the progression of such late complications into adverse health outcomes affecting quality of life.	Method: Medical record of people with Type 1 diabetes should record assessments of eye, kidney, nerve, foot, and arterial damage (all these) within the last 14 months. Measure: Percent with such assessment recorded. Method: Where evidence of eye, nerve, kidney or arterial damage is found, evidence of a plan for management of the condition within the medical record. Measure: Percent with such a plan recorded.	A record of agreed none acceptance of surveillance by the person concerned.	Eye surveillance by digital photography or examination by an ophthalmologist; kidney assessment is a measure of albumin excretion rate and serum creatinine; foot assessment includes skin condition (ulceration), sensation, foot pulses and deformity as minimum; arterial damage includes questioning on claudication, angina, and occurrence of cardiac arterial, cerebrovascular or limb arterial events. Retinal damage means any grade of retinopathy including macular change; kidney damage means albumin:creatinine ratio over 2.5 mg/mmol for men or 3.5 mg/mmol for women, or proteinuria, or creatinine >130 µmol/l; nerve

continued

Table 1: Audit criteria for key messages – *continued*

Key message	Audit criterion	Exceptions	Definition
Late complications – *continued*	*Outcome measures* Method: In people with Type 1 diabetes, prevalence of: • diabetes retinal damage • abnormality of monofilament sensory detection • abnormality of albumin excretion rate or serum creatinine • absence of both pulses in at least one foot • symptomatic angina • claudication. Measure: Statistically significant trend to improvement between years, or in best quartile when benchmarked against equivalent other services.		damage means abnormality of response to 10 g monofilament or non-traumatic pin prick (Neurotip); arterial damage means presence or experience of limb claudication, angina, cardiac vascular event, or cerebrovascular event (TIA or stroke).

THE GUIDELINE

4 Diagnosis

4.1 Rationale

The diagnosis of Type 1 diabetes would not appear to present any problems. It is, however, a lifelong condition requiring treatment with a therapy of considerable health and social impact (insulin injections) so it is important that the diagnosis is secure. Considerations also arise over differentiating the types of diabetes.

4.2 Evidence

Diagnosis, in regard of types of diabetes, is generally not addressed by the WHO report.[8] That report notes that children present with severe symptoms, and that diagnosis is simply confirmed by blood glucose measurement (advice that may be regarded as dated) (**IV**).

WHO otherwise concentrates mainly on the situation pertaining to Type 2 diabetes, in doing so noting (by reference to the 1985 report) the lack of need for challenge testing when plasma glucose levels are high in the absence of other metabolic stress, and are confirmed by a second laboratory measurement or classic symptoms.

4.3 Comment

Type 1 diabetes is, for the most part, easily recognised and diagnosed, requiring hyperglycaemia to a significant degree (risk of microvascular complications), and islet B-cell destruction which may be detected as pathogenetic markers or poor insulin secretion.

Where the diagnosis of diabetes is equivocal, and hyperglycaemia is by definition marginal, management will generally follow guidelines for Type 2 diabetes. In some patients with 'Type 2 diabetes' or diabetes of uncertain type, management will be by clinical stage even if auto-immune markers of Type 1 diabetes are detected.

If Type 1 diabetes is suspected, referral should be more urgent than with most other types of diabetes diagnosed in adults.

4.4 Consideration

The group endorsed the commentary discussed above, and concluded that simple recommendations were all that were required. Although in this condition diagnosis of diabetes is rarely in doubt, errors do arise in attribution of diabetes type on occasions, and this is known to result in negative consequences including failure to anticipate ketoacidosis or unnecessary insulin therapy. Accordingly the group felt that cautionary recommendations were in order. The group noted that formal evidence of the utility of tests to distinguish type of diabetes by auto-immune markers or measures of islet B-cell function was not positive, and that these tests were not routinely performed.

The group were keen to reiterate the importance of laboratory glucose estimation in line with WHO recommendations to avoid the very rare misdiagnoses with lifelong consequences. The role of symptoms and of HbA$_{1c}$ estimation were seen as useful but only supportive, as both lack absolute specificity.

RECOMMENDATIONS

R1   Diabetes should be confirmed by a single diagnostic laboratory glucose measurement   **D**
in the presence of classical symptoms, or by a further laboratory glucose measurement.
The diagnosis may be supported by a raised HbA$_{1c}$.

R2   Where diabetes is diagnosed, but Type 2 diabetes suspected, the diagnosis of Type 1   **D**
diabetes should be considered if:
- ketonuria is detected, or
- weight loss is marked, or
- the person does not have features of the metabolic syndrome or other contributing illness.

R3   When diabetes is diagnosed in a younger person, the possibility that the diabetes is not   **D**
Type 1 diabetes should be considered if they are obese or have a family history of diabetes,
particularly if they are of non-white ethnicity.

R4   Tests to detect specific auto-antibodies or to measure C-peptide deficiency should not   **D**
be regularly used to confirm the diagnosis of Type 1 diabetes. Their use should be
considered if predicting the rate of decline of islet B-cell function would be useful in
discriminating Type 1 from Type 2 diabetes.

5 Care process and support

5.1 Scope of this chapter

It is outside the scope of this guideline to consider service delivery issues. Accordingly no recommendations are made regarding site of care; the emphasis is on the process of care necessary for a person with Type 1 diabetes to achieve optimal yet cost-effective outcomes. For example, while it is evidence-based that multidisciplinary team care leads to a reduced rate of complications, and it is known that no health professional alone possesses all the necessary skills, no recommendation is made about the membership of multidisciplinary teams or where they are sited. Nevertheless, where an evidence base exists for an activity associated with a health professional this has been appraised (because it influences the skillmix required), even if it is not used directly in the recommendations.

Equally, a term such as 'diabetes centre' should be read as a group of people working together as a resource with access to appropriate healthcare equipment and supporting all those in the local area providing diabetes care. This should not be interpreted as buildings sited in a primary or secondary care environment, or to sole sites of care. Some items of equipment (telephones, structured records, diabetes recall registers) are necessary components for the processes of care (for example retinopathy screening) discussed in other parts of this guideline.

5.2 Optimal healthcare processes

▷ Rationale

The management of diabetes is multidimensional, and each dimension is multifaceted. Notable dimensions include diagnosis and associated management, preventative long-term care, hospital and emergency management, and detection and management of late-developing complications. With each of these dimensions a number of care areas are found (for example in long-term prevention, glucose control, blood pressure control, risk factor surveillance, blood lipid control and smoking), and for each care area a number of deliverables addressed (for example in blood glucose control: knowledge and basis of targets, injection skills, self-monitoring, dose adjustment, dietary matching, hypoglycaemia management, sick day management) by a number of different members of a multidisciplinary team. This multidimensional care delivery requirement has spawned diverse attempts aimed at ensuring optimal care is available to all those with diabetes. This section of the guideline seeks to examine what evidence is available to support some of these approaches.

▷ Evidence review

It was recognised that the systems underlying structured organisation of care (for example diabetes centres) do not easily lend themselves to comparison by higher level studies (RCTs and cohort studies). Some technologies within such systems (for example a foot care information initiative) may on occasion be so approachable, but for the most part such technologies are offered and may only be applicable as part of an integrated care package. Accordingly, for the purposes of evidence review, no limits to study type were placed on the papers sought. Of 348 titles identified, 58 were selected as relevant for critical appraisal.

Additionally the major national and international guidelines were reviewed for consistency of recommendations. As the current question was considered at the end of the guideline process, a review of generic structures of care already inherent or explicit in agreed recommendations within the current guideline was also made.

Only rarely did the primary literature distinguish type of diabetes. On occasion, insulin-treated people from both major types of diabetes were considered separately from people with Type 2 diabetes managed without insulin injections. Historically, people using insulin have been managed in specialist care; papers addressing issues of delivery of care by family doctors without reference to insulin-treated diabetes were also excluded from consideration, except in regards of complications surveillance.

▷ Evidence statements

Multidisciplinary care

The Diabetes Control and Complications Trial (DCCT),[9] and smaller RCTs using improved management to judge the effect on patient outcomes, used multidisciplinary team input (in particular from specialist nurses and dietitians) as part of an integrated package to improve metabolic intermediate outcomes. A Cochrane review[10] of diabetes specialist nurse input identified six heterogeneous studies unsuitable for meta-analysis, and found little evidence of longer-term impact on intermediate outcomes. An RCT[11] of the impact of structured team care as compared to usual care showed improved satisfaction and blood glucose control at six months. An RCT[12] of the use of diabetes specialist nurses to adjust insulin doses over the telephone showed improved blood glucose control (**Ib**).

A nurse specialist approach has been justified by a number of before-and-after studies and case series with such input[13–17] (**II**).

A number of studies of variable quality address the impact of inclusion of podiatrists compared to normal care within what is then usually called a diabetes foot care team. These studies included one RCT showing more patient knowledge and less callosities at one year, and a controlled study[18] (it is unclear whether that study is randomised) showing less foot ulceration (**Ib**).

A number of historically-controlled or descriptive studies support this approach, mainly reporting on patient preference outcomes[15,19–21] (**IV**).

The current guideline and all examined guidelines advise the use of members of a multi-disciplinary team or, more specifically, nurses with training in teaching skills and adult education in a number of aspects of patient education, and formally trained dietitians and podiatrists within the specifically relevant areas of diabetes care (**IV**).

Annual review

No RCTs address the concept of integrated annual review. Newly-implemented structured annual review has been subject to a descriptive review,[22] suggesting improved satisfaction with care and improved patient motivation. Few full-length descriptions of the review process are available,[23] most references being editorials and letters (**IV**).

The current guideline suggests annual surveillance of a number of potentially developing late complications (as do all other guidelines for the most complications). The International Diabetes Federation's European guideline recommends integration of these activities into one patient visit.[24] Annual review is also the basis of many quality control structures proposed for diabetes care,[25] including (implicitly) that of the UK Audit Commission (**IV**).

Diabetes registers

A series of descriptive papers appear to demonstrate the feasibility of establishing population-based and clinic-based diabetes registers, with varying densities of information.[26–36] A system of database-driven recall for complications surveillance is implicit in the recommendations for annual complications surveillance of this and published guidelines. Issues of data security and confidentiality are not reported to have proved to be problematic obstructions to the deployment of diabetes registers (**IV**).

Diabetes centres and structured care

Most papers in this area are descriptive, and there is inevitable overlap with deployment of multidisciplinary teams and provision of diabetes information and foot care. Using historical controls a study[37] suggests improved blood glucose control, while another non-randomised study suggests improved survival (presumably mainly in people with Type 2 diabetes) (**IIb**).

Structured records and care cards

Although papers were ascertained addressing these areas,[38–44] the papers were descriptive with no useful analysis of patient-related outcomes (**IV**).

Electronic patient records and computer data analysis

A number of descriptive papers were identified,[45–48] suggesting such approaches can be feasible and have utility, but not demonstrating comparative advantage to traditional approaches (**IV**).

However when such records were used to send judgemental letters to people with diabetes,[49] randomising sites of care, intermediate outcomes were significantly improved (probably mainly in people with Type 2 diabetes) (**Ib**).

Telemedicine

A number of approaches to medical care without direct patient contact are described in the literature. One RCT of a telecare system for insulin[50] provided equivalent control at reduced cost, while another study[12] using nurses resulted in improved blood glucose control (**Ib**).

In more rural and remote situations telemedicine can similarly provide apparent time and cost savings where images of foot problems[51] and eye photographs[52] need to be reviewed by specialists (**Ib**).

Inpatient care

Three papers using historical controls or randomised controls address the value of multidisciplinary teams with a specialist interest in diabetes management in the care of inpatients on non-diabetes wards.[53–55] Reduced length of inpatient stay is consistently reported. One study suggests improved glucose control.[55] One study, also using historical controls, addresses length of stay in a developing country in newly-diagnosed people with diabetes, showing much reduced stays with multidisciplinary team input (**Ib/IIa**).

Guidelines

No literature on the deployment or impact of diabetes guidelines was identified.

▷ Health economic evidence

Two potentially useful papers consider the type of treatment facility used to deliver care to those with Type 1 diabetes.[334,335] One German study[334] found that the treatment facility (polyclinics, specialist clinics or general practitioners) makes no difference to diabetes-specific knowledge when this was controlled for age, sex and education. One UK study[335] found no difference between hospital- and general practice-based care on a range of outcome measures for metabolic control, satisfaction with treatment or beliefs about diabetic control for a mixed diabetic population. Some differences were observed in the surveillance for complications, with more frequent testing in integrated care. Whilst costly, it is worth noting that fewer patients defaulted from general practice-based care than conventional care. Avoided complications may offset the increased cost of general practice-based care, although this cannot be established on the basis of this study.

One UK-based study[297] suggested that the provision of a hospital-based diabetes specialist nurse lowered the cost per patient admission without producing a significant difference in readmission, quality of life or patient satisfaction.

▷ Consideration

The group endorsed the approaches suggested by the evidence, but noted that attempts to implement some of the recommendations in the past had been inhibited by funding difficulties. This however was not felt to be a barrier to reiterating the health gains to be obtained. It was noted that recent publications (beyond the cut-off date of the searches) supported some of the recommendations further, including those relating to specialist nurses. The UK's national service framework for diabetes was noted to have endorsed diabetes registers. The group recognised the lack of any kind of formal evidence relating to walk-in, telephone-request and out-of-hours services.

RECOMMENDATIONS

R5   Advice to adults with Type 1 diabetes should be provided by a range of professionals   **D**
with skills in diabetes care working together in a coordinated approach. A common environment (diabetes centre) is an important resource in allowing a diabetes multidisciplinary team to work and communicate efficiently while providing consistent advice.

R6   Open access services should be provided on a walk-in and telephone-request basis   C
during working hours to adults with Type 1 diabetes, and a helpline staffed by people
with specific diabetes expertise should be provided on a 24-hour basis. Adults with
diabetes should be provided with contact information for these services.

R7   An individual care plan should be set up and reviewed annually, modified according to   D
changes in wishes, circumstances and medical findings, and the details recorded. The
plan should include aspects of:
- diabetes education including nutritional advice (see section 6.1, 'Education
  programmes for adults with Type 1 diabetes' and 6.3, 'Dietary management')
- insulin therapy (see section 7.3, 'Insulin regimens' and 7.4, 'Insulin delivery')
- self-monitoring (see section 6.2, 'Self-monitoring of blood glucose')
- arterial risk factor surveillance and management (see chapter 8, 'Arterial risk control')
- late complications surveillance and management (see sections on late complications)
- means and frequency of communication with the professional care team
- follow-up consultations including next annual review.

R8   Population, practice-based and clinic diabetes registers (as specified by the national   D
service framework) should be used to assist programmed recall for annual review and
assessment of complications and vascular risk.

R9   Conventional technology (telephones), or newer technologies for high-density data   A
transmission of images, should be used to improve process and outcomes.

R10   The multidisciplinary team approach should be available to inpatients with Type 1   D
diabetes, regardless of the reason for admission (see section 13.3, 'Inpatient management').

5.3   Support groups

▷ Rationale

As having Type 1 diabetes can have a major impact on lifestyle and self-esteem, it would appear
that support groups could have a role in providing for some needs outside the professional
environment and even separately from immediate carers. The range of such potential input is
large and might stretch from simply fulfilling a need for belonging, through to helping with
diabetes-related financial problems (such as insurance), and even providing a further source of
diabetes-related information.

Coping with diabetes, or any other condition, is influenced not only by psychological
characteristics of the individual but also by social relationships (eg support and communication
by healthcare team, family and friends). Informal interpersonal variables, such as social
resources and support, have been found to be associated with better diabetes self-management,[56–7] family environment,[58–60] and marital interaction.[61] A medical condition is only one
aspect that affects the make-up of an individual's personal identity, and for some may be
perceived as a minor factor compared to their environmental and social circumstances.

A 'support group' is defined in this guideline as a group of people with Type 1 diabetes that
comes together to provide support to themselves and others in their locality. Members are
usually unpaid and many will be supported under the auspices of national (or local) voluntary
organisations. Support groups have become commonplace throughout health and social care.

Patients and carers may choose to contact or be involved with support groups to gain information and support to benefit their own needs, or with a wider altruistic aim of helping other people within the local community. It was not possible to find specific research identifying patient and carer preferences for support groups, or indeed to identify specific groups or types of people who may benefit more than others. Some people attend meetings of groups regularly whilst other individuals are reassured by being aware of a group's existence and the opportunity to contact the group at a later date if problems arise and/or support is required. Preferences are dependent on what stage people are at in their lives and what information is taken (or needs to be taken) on board.

▷ Evidence statements

The Diabetes Attitudes, Wishes and Needs (DAWN) questionnaire study[62] highlighted that emotional support, along with family support, was a key factor in how well people with diabetes manage their condition, with support networks being considered at least as important as the medication they take in helping them manage their diabetes. Interim results also indicate that people who do not have access to a community of support, especially the young or elderly living alone, may be less likely to be concordant with their medication regimes, putting them at risk of inadequate control of their diabetes (III).

There are still significant numbers of people emerging from the confirmation of a diagnosis who are underinformed and unsupported.[63] Qualitative research of various designs examining the views and experiences of people with diabetes and carers has identified that many perceived benefits exist from meeting other people with diabetes. It has helped many to overcome the feelings of isolation and is seen as an opportunity to talk to others going through the same experience[64] (IV).

Research evaluating the effectiveness of support groups for patients and carers, across numerous conditions and groups (not necessarily diabetes), has shown specific benefits including (III):

- psychological and emotional benefits[65] including lower pain perception and improved ability to cope with stress[63,66–7]
- reduction of carers' burdens and stresses[68–9]
- improvement in quality of life[70–71]
- improved self-care through health promotion strategies which have been helpful in smoking cessation and management of chronic conditions[72–3]
- improved access to health service provision[74]
- reduced isolation, overcoming depression and loss of self-esteem[64]
- better understanding of conditions, symptoms and healthcare systems through education and information.[67]

The Diabetes UK network of support groups recorded 175,426 members in July 2003, with around 7% under the age of 20 years and around 30% aged 70 years or over. Around 40% had paid for annual adult membership, 50% had a reduced rate membership (including children), and 10% had chosen life membership. The Diabetes UK Careline is, at the time of writing, one of the busiest sources of information for all people with Type 1 diabetes in the UK. In 2002, Careline were contacted 40,747 times (81% telephone, 13% e-mail, 6% post).

The five most frequent topics of enquiry recorded were (III):[67a]

- diet
- insulin
- medicines other than insulin
- new diagnosis
- travel.

▷ Health economic evidence

Two studies were identified as potentially useful in this area.[336-7] As neither paper included cost information, the cost-effectiveness of support interventions cannot be ascertained.

RECOMMENDATION

R11   At the time of diagnosis and periodically thereafter, adults with Type 1 diabetes should   C
       be offered up-to-date information on the existence of and means of contacting diabetes
       support groups (local and national) and the benefits of membership.

5.4   Quality audit and monitoring

▷ Rationale

It is generally accepted now that any system delivering a product, including healthcare systems, can benefit from review of its performance. The diabetes care espoused by this guideline is both complex and systematic, and thus lends itself to the kind of data collection needed for quality development. That very complexity, however, means that monitoring the structures, process and outcomes of all sectors can seem overwhelming, necessitating consideration of how limited monitoring activity can be undertaken without distorting the areas gaining attention for improvement. Monitoring of quality of life would seem *a priori* to be of particular importance in diabetes care, but presents its own difficulties of data acquisition and of analysis of temporally different outcomes.

Audit criteria are suggested in section 3.3 of this guideline to assist local users in promoting implementation and monitoring ongoing improvements in process and outcome. They have been informed where possible by existing validated measures, principally those of the National Centre for Health Outcome Development.[75]

6 | Education progammes and self-care

6.1 Education programmes for adults with Type 1 diabetes

▷ Rationale

Having diabetes involves acquiring a great range of new skills and knowledge, including insulin therapy, dietary changes, self-monitoring, hypoglycaemia, jobs, travel, physical exercise, coping with concurrent illness, foot care, arterial risk control and avoiding complications. The history of education and information giving in diabetes care goes back to the earliest dietary interventions several centuries ago, and the use of education professionals to impart skills associated with insulin therapy dates from the time of discovery and isolation of insulin. Accordingly patient education is a true cornerstone that enables self-management of diabetes, and most diabetes management is self-management. Review of other parts of this NICE guideline will reveal that education and information giving are parts of nearly all of them, from enabling patient choice in determining features of self-management, to acquisition of skills needed to perform tasks and make judgements, to self-care where high risk complications have developed, and to skills in handling healthcare professionals to ensure that issues of importance to the person with Type 1 diabetes are addressed.

▷ Evidence statements

Content of education

There were no trials located in newly-diagnosed people with Type 1 diabetes specifically, or concerned with the initial content of education. The American Diabetes Association (ADA) guidelines[76] suggest that as part of initial visit people should be referred to a diabetes educator if education is not provided by the physician or practice staff, but content of this education is not defined (**IV**).

Educational setting

One small randomised controlled trial[77] comparing the efficacy of classroom teaching of diabetes skills, compared to individualised learning, found that classroom teaching led to a greater level of awareness about diabetes self-care. However, there was no significant difference in terms of the level of use of self-care practices. Furthermore, the two education techniques provided no different outcome of levels of technical skill in self-care. However this study made no analysis of comparability of study groups at baseline and was not blinded (**Ib**).

Technology interventions

One randomised controlled study compared two interactive computer schemes to reinforce an educational video. The first gave additional feedback and information on the correct answers, the second only the correct answers.[78] People with diabetes in the interactive group scored significantly better in a follow-up test of diabetes knowledge than those following the standard scheme. There were no significant differences in user ratings for the two software packages, but the people in the additional feedback group had a better diabetes knowledge at baseline, so the results may be biased by this confounding factor (**Ib**).

Guidelines for self-management education

An update of the US standards for diabetes self-management education[79] based on a literature review covered the organisation of diabetes self-management education, its content and provision. A multiprofessional task force encompassing all the major interested stakeholders agreed the following standards (**IV**).

❑ Education and information-giving will involve the interaction of the individual with diabetes with a multifaceted education instructional team, which may include a behaviourist, exercise physiologist, ophthalmologist, optometrist, pharmacist, physician, podiatrist, registered dietitian, registered nurse, other healthcare professionals, and paraprofessionals.

❑ Instructors will obtain regular continuing education in the areas of diabetes management, behavioural interventions, teaching and learning skills and counselling skills.

❑ Assessed needs of the individual will determine which of the following content areas are delivered:
   – describing the diabetes disease process and treatment options
   – incorporating appropriate nutritional management
   – incorporating physical activity into lifestyle
   – utilising medications (if applicable) for therapeutic effectiveness
   – monitoring blood glucose and urine ketones (where appropriate) and using results to improve control
   – preventing, detecting and treating acute complications
   – preventing (through risk reduction behaviour), detecting and treating chronic complications
   – goal-setting to promote health, and problem-solving for daily living
   – integrating psychosocial adjustment to daily life
   – promoting preconception care, management during pregnancy and gestational diabetes management (if applicable).

❑ An individualised assessment, development of an education plan and periodic reassessment between participant and instructor will direct the selection of appropriate educational materials and interventions.

❑ The assessment includes relevant medical history, cultural influences, health beliefs and attitudes, diabetes knowledge, self-management skills and behaviours, readiness to learn, cognitive ability, physical limitations, family support and financial status.

❑ There shall be documentation of the individual's assessment, education plan, intervention, evaluation and follow-up in the permanent confidential education record.

General education programmes

Within an overall review of patient education models for diabetes (not type-specific) one health technology assessment[80] reviewing four controlled trials of a range of education programmes including items of self-management, self-monitoring, diet and the effects of insulin and exercise, taught by a variety of staff or self-taught, and as an initial intense course or as ongoing programmes, reported a variety of positive outcomes compared to normal care. This review found that one study had demonstrated improvements over 10 years in diabetic control, in terms of reduced HbA$_{1c}$ levels. In another study, an intensive five-day training course was found to be effective in reducing HbA$_{1c}$ levels. In one study there was no difference in blood glucose control with education compared to usual care, while there were no between-group comparisons made in another other study. Education was also shown to improve blood pressure. There is limited evidence to suggest a reduced rate of ketoacidosis and reduced hospitalisation. However, there was no evidence to indicate that education can reduce body mass index. There is some data to suggest increased incidence of hypoglycaemic episodes. Long-term outcomes of retinopathy or neuropathy were not found to be significantly affected by education, but there is some limited evidence to suggest nephropathy incidence is improved, although rates were low. Unsurprisingly, diabetes knowledge was significantly improved with education, although this was not true of quality of life. Overall the included trials were of moderate methodological rigour. Three of the trials included were investigating education in the context of intensification of treatment compared to normal care, and it is difficult to be sure that the benefits reported are directly attributable to the education aspect of the intervention (**NICE**).

Metabolic control and quality of life were not found to be significantly affected by a structured outpatient programme of education led by a nurse, dietitian and other people with diabetes over four weeks in a large randomised trial as compared to conventional care[81] (**Ib**).

A medium-sized randomised controlled trial[82] of a monthly education programme at which different aspects of diabetes treatment and technical skills were considered found that after one year of education HbA$_{1c}$ levels were reduced compared with normal clinical care in people with Type 1 diabetes. However, age differences between the control and intervention groups at baseline mean that this study is possibly methodologically limited (**Ib**).

Another moderate-sized systematic review of eight trials encompassing over 3,000 patients with either Type 1 or Type 2 diabetes,[83] found that intensive *vs* brief education on foot care provided a significant decrease in incidence of foot ulcers, and in one trial amputations, but no difference in the same outcomes over seven years in another study. This is despite three trials reporting successful uptake of messages regarding foot care behaviour. Another trial reported in this review found that an intensive educational intervention including both people with diabetes and doctors improved the prevalence of serious foot lesions compared to usual care, although the composite outcome of all foot lesions and amputations was not significantly improved. Authors of the review noted methodological limitations of the included studies, and outcome reporting times varied between individual trials (**Ia**).

Diabetes self-management education

Evaluation, in a large systematic review,[84] of a range of diabetes self-management education (DSME) programmes compared to normal routine levels in populations of people with diabetes found that interventions based in community gathering places were able to reduce blood glycated haemoglobin (GHb) and fasting blood glucose levels. There is some evidence that they can also improve diabetes knowledge and improve physical activity (minutes of walking). Other trials reviewed that were based in the home setting – half of which included children or adolescents – showed a significant decrease in GHb after DSME, and a borderline beneficial effect on weight for people undergoing DSME as compared to conventional care. Specific analysis in patients with Type 1 diabetes found no significant change in diabetes knowledge with such programmes (**Ia**).

Other educational interventions

A small randomised controlled trial[12] in people with Type 1 diabetes found that an intervention whereby patients received regular telephone contact with a diabetes nurse to alter insulin regimen decreased HbA_{1c} over six months compared to usual care. This difference was not found to be affected by age, sex or type of diabetes (**Ib**).

Behavioural and education interventions

There are no systematic reviews and few prospective randomised studies that report on methods to improve concordance in self-management in people with Type 1 diabetes. One small unblinded study,[85] which was methodologically limited owing to high drop-out rates and inequalities in patient characteristics at baseline, found that an intervention of a self-taught study programme to improve self-control behaviour was able to demonstrate improved adherence to goals of self-monitoring of blood glucose level over 12 weeks. The intervention included a wide range of educational and behavioural choice items, and the relative effectiveness of any of these is hard to define. The methodological limitations of the study would not form a rigorous basis for recommending such an approach (**Ib**).

A similar intervention among adolescents (mean age 18 years) in India enrolled in a prospective randomised trial,[86] with an intervention of 15 hours of individualised learning over three months comprising both behavioural and cognitive strategies based on an operant learning model, found improved adherence on a composite three-item scale, compared to usual care. This improved adherence was mirrored in significantly improved blood glucose level compared to people in the control group. However, this study had a small sample size and was unblinded, and it was not possible to determine whether benefits persist after the cessation of the intervention (**Ib**).

Education interventions

One small- to medium-sized randomised trial of a specialist education programme delivered to people with Type 1 diabetes by a team of physicians, dietitians and specialist nurses found there to be no statistically significant differences in diabetes knowledge or adherence to dietary advice compared to a control group who received conventional diabetes education. Both groups improved in both measures immediately after the completion of the education intervention but then knowledge and adherence fell away with time. This trial was sited in Finland and there may be differences in content of conventional diabetes education compared to that of the UK care setting[87] (**Ib**).

Monitoring devices

There were no significant differences in adherence to glucose self-monitoring or in blood glucose levels reported at six months between two interventions with novel glucose monitoring devices and control with a standard device from a medium-sized multicentre randomised trial.[88] The trial included a population of people with Type 1 diabetes who had had the condition for an average of 14 years. The study was blinded between the two novel monitoring machines, but the people in the control group would have been aware that they were not receiving the intervention as they continued to use their usual machine. To evaluate adherence all patients were asked to keep diaries of self-monitoring behaviour and this may have stimulated greater adherence even in the control group than under normal everyday self-monitoring conditions (**Ib**).

▷ Health economic evidence

Assessing the cost-effectiveness of patient education is complicated by the fact that patient education is rarely assessed in isolation. Recent NICE guidance[338] into patient education models considered the health economic evidence for interventions in terms of self-care, quality of life and the long-term complications of diabetes. Interventions improving knowledge of diabetes were excluded from consideration, as improved knowledge of diabetes does not necessarily affect subsequent outcomes.

The NICE appraisal found only two published health economic papers suitable for assessing patient education.[339,340] Of these, only one[339] included Type 1 diabetes patients, and this established cost-effectiveness ratios for altering food habits.

▷ Consideration

The group noted that patient education was a necessary and logical part of most aspects of diabetes self-care, and that self-care was a social, health and economic necessity in the management of the condition. Specific recommendations related to aspects of care such as self-monitoring, insulin therapy, foot care and nutrition were thought best presented in the individual sections of this guideline. The group noted inappropriateness of the classical clinical trial model when just one feature of an integrated package was varied, and one of many possible outputs monitored as primary outcome. There is also the difficulty of, and lack of funding for, the larger, longer-term trials used for pharmaceutical interventions. Equally, the central role of education in achieving success in blood glucose control and health outcomes (DCCT and other key studies) could not be ignored. Such information suggested that educational interventions were likely to be cost-effective, but it was impossible to make comparative judgements of different education models, a conclusion seemingly also reached by the NICE Appraisal Committee on the basis of a report from the University of Southampton's health technology assessment unit.

Issues of information overload at the stressful time of diagnosis, the size of the longer-term educational needs of individuals, the diversity of individual needs, and the retention of the information needed to make informed choices, and the group's experience of these in practice, served to guide recommendations broadly in line with those of Diabetes UK and the International Diabetes Federation (Europe).

RECOMMENDATIONS

Specific recommendations on patient education and information-giving in particular aspects of care are given in individual sections of this guideline.

R12   A programme of structured diabetes education covering all major aspects of diabetes self-care and the reasons for it should be made available to all adults with Type 1 diabetes in the months after diagnosis, and periodically thereafter according to agreed need following yearly assessment.   A

R13   Education programmes for adults with Type 1 diabetes should be flexible so that they can be adapted to specific educational, social and cultural needs. These needs should be integrated with individual health needs as dictated by the impact of diabetes and other relevant health conditions on the individual.   D

R14   Education programmes for adults with Type 1 diabetes should be designed and delivered by members of the multidisciplinary diabetes team in accordance with the principles of adult education.   D

R15   Education programmes for adults with Type 1 diabetes should include modules designed to empower adults to participate in their own healthcare through: D
- enabling them to make judgements and choices about how they effect that care
- obtaining appropriate input from the professionals available to advise them.

R16   Professionals engaged in the delivery of diabetes care should consider incorporating educational interchange at all opportunities when in contact with a person with Type 1 diabetes. The professional should have the skills and training to make best use of such time.   D

R17   More formal review of self-care and needs should be made annually in all adults with Type 1 diabetes, and the agenda addressed each year should vary according to the priorities agreed between the healthcare professional and the person with Type 1 diabetes.   D

6.2   Self-monitoring of blood glucose

▷   Rationale

Insulin therapy has to be adjusted with lifestyle, insulin dose requirements vary from individual to individual, and the effects of insulin injections are notoriously erratic. It might seem obvious that being able to keep an hour-to-hour or day-to-day check on actual blood glucose levels would be to the advantage of any person using insulin therapy. Potential should exist here to assist with diabetes self-education, dose optimisation, reassurance over hypoglycaemia and helping professionals give optimum advice on insulin regimens.

▷   Evidence statements

Reliability and validity

Papers contained within a systematic review[89] suggest that the evidence on issues of observer training, interdevice variability, the effects of long-term use and patient acceptability have not been adequately addressed (**IV**).

Table 2 Some appropriate content of education programmes for people with Type 1 diabetes and those personally involved with helping in their day-to-day care*

Around time of diagnosis

- ❏ The aims of management and outcome of good self-management
- ❏ Self-injection and self-monitoring skills
- ❏ Nutritional information for people on insulin injection therapy
- ❏ Detection and management of hypoglycaemia
- ❏ Establishing healthy lifestyle

In the period following diagnosis

- ❏ Reinforcement of above
- ❏ Use of professional advisors and the healthcare system
- ❏ Integration of flexible eating and insulin dosing
- ❏ Goals of self-management
- ❏ Long-term risks and their amelioration (including arterial risk)
- ❏ Management of intercurrent illness and developing complications
- ❏ Role of preventative therapeutic interventions, side effects and importance
- ❏ Lifestyle issues including employment, travel (including across time zones), driving
- ❏ Contraception, pregnancy and children

In the longer term

- ❏ Self-care of late complications including foot care
- ❏ Reinforcement based on annual review of need

See also the recommendations of IDF (Europe)[24] and Diabetes UK.[282]

One study within the systematic review[89] comparing self-reported readings against a memory meter showed that inaccuracies in readings were common. This was due to rounding of values, omission of outlying values and reporting of results when no test had been performed. These findings were confirmed in another reviewed study of 14 people who recorded lower blood glucose values in logbook records than meter memories (**Ia**).

Reported within the systematic review, one trial[89] suggested that patients needed to be informed of the memory capacity of their meters to improve accuracy. A further study reported in the review argued that the true diurnal variability in glycaemia in people with Type 1 diabetes is too great to be measured, even when self-monitoring of blood glucose (SMBG) is repeated seven times daily (**Ia**).

Patient factors (as described below) were shown to have an impact (both positive and negative) on the reliability of monitoring in five studies.[89]

Reliability can be improved through proper training of patients, and was shown in sub-group analysis to be equally as good in older people, and people with visual impairments (on condition that extensive instruction has been provided).

One study concluded that impairment of colour vision affects the ability to interpret self-monitoring with visually read strips, suggesting that all patients should be screened for colour vision before self-monitoring begins (**Ia**).

Clinical effectiveness of blood glucose monitoring

Four trials contained within a systematic review[89] failed to show with sufficient power a demonstrated effect of SMBG on blood glucose control (**Ia**).

Two trials comparing urine and blood testing showed no clinical difference in the two tests[89] (**Ia**).

A systematic review[89] reported on patient preferences for different monitoring techniques. One trial reported patients preferring blood testing, or a combination of blood and urine testing, compared to urine testing alone. No preference was stated for visual strips or strips with meters (**Ia**).

One methodologically-limited crossover study[90] comparing blood glucose meters with visual test strips showed patients found the two techniques equally convenient to use, although overall more patients preferred the blood glucose meter.

Preferences were based on: accuracy, confidence in test result, no judgement by patient, inability to cheat with result and use of the built in timer (**Ib**).

One methodologically-limited comparative study[91] showed that fructosamine self-test results correlated well with laboratory test with very low bias. Imprecision of the self-test was higher than the laboratory test, but could still identify patients with good *vs* poor glycaemic control (**DS**).

A further methodologically-limited diagnostic study[92] in people with Type 2 diabetes showed self-testing of fructosamine to be comparable in accuracy to laboratory fructosamine and GHb values (**CDS**).

One trial with 25 patients[93] showed no significant difference in glucose control or patient practice based on frequency of testing. The authors stated that they are unable to identify any optimal frequency for blood glucose self-monitoring in typical diabetic population. There is little or no relationship between the frequency of blood glucose monitoring, the frequency of insulin dose adjustments and the level of metabolic control (**Ib**).

A study of the preferences of 18 patients within a systematic review[89] reported a preference for testing four times daily twice weekly, or four times daily once a week, compared to twice daily every day of the week (**Ib**).

One study from a systematic review reported fasting plasma glucose to be less useful as an accurate mode of monitoring in insulin-treated people with diabetes than in other people[89] (**IIa**).

▷ Health economic evidence

The DCCT included self-monitoring of blood glucose as part of intensive treatment. Self-monitoring is only likely to have an effect on blood glucose control when used to inform the management of diabetes. As such, it is not feasible to analyse its cost-effectiveness in isolation from the requirements of subsequent management strategies.

A recent HTA report[89] identifies one paper considering the cost-effectiveness of blood or urine glucose monitoring against 'conventional dietary control' amongst those with Type 1 diabetes.[341] This paper is based on Russian conditions and also includes education in the intervention technologies. The GDG felt that differences in international healthcare systems mean little weight could be placed on its assertions that no significant difference exists between blood and urine glucose monitoring.

▷ Consideration

Self-monitoring does not, in itself, appear to improve blood glucose control. However, the group noted that it was an essential component of the markedly improved blood glucose control with improved outcomes demonstrated in the landmark DCCT study, and indeed in the other smaller studies of blood glucose control and complications. Indeed it was difficult for members of the group to conceive how modern flexible insulin dosage regimens could be adopted without it. However, the technique is not easy, painless or convenient, and as a result no one system is found appropriate for use by all individuals. Improved technical facility could be identified from clinical experience. Nevertheless appropriate training and quality of skills review is agreed as necessary and normal practice. Different individuals are noted to use this technology with different frequencies and for different needs according to personal preferences. Given the nature of the technology it is rarely abused.

A newer approach, using smaller blood samples from non-finger-prick sites, was not judged to have adequate evidence of reliability, particularly in the situation of hypoglycaemia, to allow a general recommendation.

RECOMMENDATIONS

R18   Self-monitoring of blood glucose levels should be used as part of an integrated package   D
that includes appropriate insulin regimens and education to help choice and
achievement of optimal diabetes outcomes.

R19   Self-monitoring skills should be taught close to the time of diagnosis and initiation   D
of insulin therapy.

R20   Self-monitoring results should be interpreted in the light of clinically significant life   D
events.

R21   Self-monitoring should be performed using meters and strips chosen by adults with   D
Type 1 diabetes to suit their needs, and usually with low blood requirements, fast
analysis times and integral memories.

R22   Structured assessment of self-monitoring skills, the quality and use made of the results   D
obtained and the equipment used should be made annually. Self-monitoring skills
should be reviewed as part of annual review or, more frequently, according to need and
reinforced where appropriate.

R23   Adults with Type 1 diabetes should be advised that the optimal frequency of   D
self-monitoring will depend on:
- the characteristics of their blood glucose control

- the insulin treatment regimen
- personal preference in using the results to achieve the desired lifestyle.

R24   Adults with Type 1 diabetes should be advised that the optimal targets for short-term   **D**
glycaemic control are:
- a pre-prandial blood glucose level of 4.0–7.0 mmol/l and
- a post-prandial blood glucose level of less than 9.0 mmol/l.

Note: These values are different to those given in the recommendations for children and young people with Type 1 diabetes because of clinical differences between these two age groups.

R25   Monitoring using sites other than the finger tips (often the forearm, using meters that   **D**
require small volumes of blood and devices to obtain those small volumes) cannot be recommended as a routine alternative to conventional self-blood glucose monitoring.

6.3   Dietary management

▷   Rationale

The imperfect nature of insulin replacement therapy, and in particular the prospective, erratic and inappropriate profiles of insulin absorption, make it necessary to understand the effects of different foods on glucose excursions if these excursions are to be appropriately minimised. Furthermore, people with Type 1 diabetes are at high arterial risk, which might be ameliorated by appropriate nutritional choices, while some associated conditions can be partly managed through nutritional advice.

▷   Evidence statements

Changes to diet

Four small randomised controlled trials[94–97] were identified examining different diet regimens in people with Type 1 diabetes. One randomised controlled study[94] found that a high fibre diet (50 g/day) for 24 weeks compared to a low fibre diet (15 g/day) improved blood glucose profile, and number of hypoglycaemic events, although HbA_{1c}, cholesterol, body weight and insulin dose were not affected (**Ib**).

A high carbohydrate, high fibre and low fat diet, compared to conventional low carbohydrate diet, taught by a dietitian in an unblinded randomised controlled trial[97] was seen at 12 months to improve HbA_{1c} (**Ib**).

The addition of vitamin E to the normal diet has been shown to provide no benefit in terms of cholesterol level, HbA_{1c}, body mass index (BMI), insulin dose or blood pressure over a 12-month period[96] (**Ib**).

There were significant improvements in glomerular filtration rate, and a decline in albuminuria after four weeks of a low protein diet compared to a normal protein diet in a randomised prospective trial in people with overt diabetic nephropathy.[95] Outcomes of urinary sodium excretion, blood pressure, BMI and HbA_{1c} were not significantly different between the diets (**Ib**).

Therapy adjustment for normal eating

Canadian clinical practice guidelines[98] recommend that all people with diabetes on fixed-dose insulin regimen should have an individualised meal and activity plan developed. Two studies showed that patients should be taught how to adjust insulin dosage, diet and physical activity in response to blood glucose levels to reduce incidence of hypoglycaemia (**Ia**).

A medium-sized randomised controlled trial[99] of a five-day outpatient programme to enable patients to replace insulin by matching it to desired carbohydrate intake amongst adults with Type 1 diabetes found that the intervention improved HbA_{1c} compared to a control of normal care to six months. Positive effects were also seen in weighted quality of life and total well-being. There was no effect on incidence of severe hypoglycaemia, weight or total cholesterol. This trial enrolled people with poorly-controlled diabetes (**Ib**).

A similar small trial[96] in which intensified insulin plus simplified diet was compared to conventional therapy and diet found HbA_{1c} to be significantly reduced, although there was no differences between the study groups for outcomes of body weight, BMI, cholesterol or triglycerides (**Ib**).

Undefined diet

A large cohort study[100] comparing degree of liberalisation of diet away from a specific controlled diet after a treatment and teaching programme with estimation of carbohydrate intake and subsequent insulin self-adjustment found that there was no significant relationship between BMI and degree of diet liberalisation. In addition there was no relationship with HbA_{1c} level or severe hypoglycaemia. However there was a relationship between liberalised diet and higher cholesterol levels, and an inverse relationship with tendency to monitor blood glucose more than three times a day (**IIa**).

Other evidence

The recent evidence-based guidelines for nutrition principles developed by the ADA,[76] provide a broad overview of research in the area of improved diabetes care for people with Type 1 diabetes through beneficial nutritional therapies. There are recommendations based on well-performed RCTs showing significant effectiveness of interventions for areas such as carbohydrates, dietary fat, energy balance and obesity, nutritional therapy for the treatment or prevention of acute complications, and hypertension. Recommendations in other key areas are based on cohort or uncontrolled studies (**Ia**).

▷ Health economic evidence

The recent NICE Technology Appraisal[101] into patient education models (**www.nice. org.uk/cat.asp?c=68326**) recommends dose adjustment for normal eating (DAFNE), and the intensified treatment required by DAFNE, as cost effective.

▷ Consideration

The group was impressed by the systematic approach to nutritional recommendations published by the ADA,[76] and the consistency of that approach with the new recommendations from Diabetes UK.[107] Consideration of the existing guidelines in the area did not lead the group to any divergent recommendations on nutrition. Furthermore, recent NICE guidance on education models for people with Type 1 diabetes had particularly addressed the relevance of one programme for mealtime insulin dose adjustment (DAFNE) and, after due discussion of some of the issues surrounding that study including the health economic issues, it was felt inappropriate to recommend modification of any of the appraisal's conclusions. Accordingly the recommendations agreed by the group are mainly those of emphasis and approach appropriate to people with Type 1 diabetes, but reflecting both management of blood glucose excursions and arterial risk.

RECOMMENDATIONS

R26   Nutritional information sensitive to personal needs and culture should be offered from the time of diagnosis of Type 1 diabetes.   **D**

R27   Nutritional information should be offered individually and as part of a diabetes education programme (see 'Patient Education' recommendations in this chapter (R12-17). Information should include advice from professionals with specific and approved training and continuing accredited education in delivering nutritional advice to people with health conditions. Opportunities to receive nutritional advice should be offered at intervals agreed between adults with Type 1 diabetes and their advising professionals.   **D**

R28   The hyperglycaemic effects of different foods a person with Type 1 diabetes wishes to eat should be discussed in the context of the insulin preparations chosen to match those food choices.   **A**

R29   Programmes should be available to adults with Type 1 diabetes to enable them to make: **A**
- optimal choices about the variety of foods they wish to consume
- insulin dose changes appropriate to reduce glucose excursions when taking different quantities of those foods.

R30   The choice of content, timing and amount of snacks between meals or at bedtime available to the person with Type 1 diabetes should be agreed on the basis of informed discussion about the extent and duration of the effects of consumption of different food types and the insulin preparations available to match them. Those choices should be modified on the basis of discussion of the results of self-monitoring tests.   **D**

R31   Information should also be made available on: **D**
- effects of different alcohol-containing drinks on blood glucose excursions and calorie intake
- use of high calorie and high sugar 'treats'
- use of foods of high glycaemic index.

R32   Information about the benefits of healthy eating in reducing arterial risk should be   D
made available as part of dietary education in the period after diagnosis, and according
to need and interest at intervals thereafter. This should include information about low
glycaemic index foods, fruit and vegetables, and types and amounts of fat, and ways of
making the appropriate nutritional changes.

R33   Nutritional recommendations to individuals should be modified to take account of   D
associated features of diabetes, including:
- excess weight and obesity
- underweight
- eating disorders
- raised blood pressure
- renal failure.

R34   All healthcare professionals providing advice on the management of Type 1 diabetes   D
should be aware of appropriate nutritional advice on common topics of concern and
interest to adults living with Type 1 diabetes, and should be prepared to seek advice from
colleagues with more specialised knowledge. Suggested common topics include:
- glycaemic index of specific foods
- body weight, energy balance and obesity management
- cultural and religious diets, feasts and fasts
- foods sold as 'diabetic'
- sweeteners
- dietary fibre intake
- protein intake
- vitamin and mineral supplements
- alcohol
- matching carbohydrate, insulin and physical activity
- salt intake in hypertension
- co-morbidities including nephropathy and renal failure, coeliac disease, cystic fibrosis or
  eating disorders
- use of peer support groups.

6.4   Physical activity

▷   Rationale

Many people wish to perform varying amounts of physical exercise, but this can interact to
disturb blood glucose levels in people on insulin therapy. Physical exercise is usually
recommended to the general population as part of a package of lifestyle measures to improve
future health, in particular reduction of arterial risk, which is markedly elevated in people with
Type 1 diabetes.

▷ Evidence statements

Aerobic exercise

One small randomised controlled trial[102] was identified that assessed the effect of a 16-week aerobic exercise programme on fitness and lipid profile in young men with Type 1 diabetes. There were significant differences in VO_{2max} and serum total cholesterol compared to no training. There were no significant changes in outcomes of HbA_{1c} and plasma glucose. The study was not blinded due to the nature of the intervention (**Ib**).

A small cross-sectional study[103] evaluating the effect of three months of individualised aerobic exercise in altering blood pressure and lipid profile found that HbA_{1c}, fructosamine and total blood glucose did not change significantly from baseline levels. The design of the study would not represent a sound basis for supporting a recommendation for advocating exercise as therapy (**IIa**).

Another study with a similar intervention[102] found that four months of aerobic training provided no changes in terms of HbA_{1c} or total cholesterol, although there were benefits of exercise compared to control in terms of peak oxygen uptake (**IIb**).

A prospective non-randomised study[104] with a before and after design found that steady-state plasma glucose was significantly decreased compared to baseline as was plasma insulin with supervised exercise program (at least 135 minutes/week) for three months compared to no exercise. Also cholesterol decreased significantly, however there were no reported significant changes in fasting blood glucose, HbA_{1c} and microalbuminuria (**IIb**).

Education and exercise

A medium-sized randomised controlled trial[105] of intensive advice and lifestyle programme with specified diet and exercise prescriptions compared to conventional care found that HbA_{1c} decreased from baseline measurements significantly over six months in the control group but remained relatively stable in the intervention group, but no between-group comparison was made. Also, HDL cholesterol and triglycerides were not significantly different between groups at any phase of the study. However exercise sessions were not standardised in the study and a lack of blinding limited the validity of the trial (**Ib**).

A small before and after study[106] found that an intervention of 10 hours of education and physical training three or four times a week produced no metabolic response at three months with fasting plasma glucose levels and serum cholesterol not changing significantly. Without blinding or randomisation this evidence is not sufficient to support the use of a mixed education and exercise intervention for people with Type 1 diabetes (**IIb**).

Other exercise

A non-randomised prospective controlled study[103] to assess whether exercise is related to better diabetes control was reviewed. There was no significant correlation between the exercise expenditure and HbA_{1c} in all Type 1 diabetes patients, nor was there any relationship to the frequency of mild hypoglycaemic events (**IIa**).

Guidelines on exercise

The ADA[76] guidelines present recommendations based on a good evidence-based review. They recommend that a thorough evaluation be undertaken of patients before exercise is initiated. General recommendations for how to exercise safely include:

- metabolic control before activity
- blood glucose monitoring before and after physical activity
- food intake to be considered with added carbohydrate as necessary (**Ia**).

▷ Health economic evidence

No evidence was found on the cost-effectiveness of programmes encouraging physical activity for Type 1 diabetes.

▷ Consideration

The group noted that the evidence for an improved arterial risk profile in people with Type 1 diabetes was consistent with that for other diabetic and non-diabetic people. Evidence of a consistent effect in improving blood glucose control was absent, although by analogy with people with Type 2 diabetes the overweight/insulin-resistant person might benefit from an exercise programme as part of a lifestyle improvement initiative. Some people will undertake significant exercise by choice and would benefit from support in so doing.

RECOMMENDATIONS

R35   Adults with Type 1 diabetes should be advised that physical activity can reduce their enhanced arterial risk in the medium and longer term.   C

R36   Adults with Type 1 diabetes who choose to integrate increased physical activity into a more healthy lifestyle should be offered information about: D
- appropriate intensity and frequency of physical activity
- role of self-monitoring of changed insulin and/or nutritional needs
- effect of activity on blood glucose levels (a fall is likely) when insulin levels are adequate
- effect of exercise on blood glucose levels when hyperglycaemic and hypoinsulinaemic (risk of worsening of hyperglycaemia and ketonaemia)
- appropriate adjustments of insulin dosage and/or nutritional intake for exercise and post-exercise periods, and the next 24 hours
- interactions of exercise and alcohol
- further contacts and sources of information.

6.5   Cultural and individual lifestyle

▷ Rationale

Cultural and genetic differences between ethnic groups are known to affect health and response to healthcare for many diseases. In regard of Type 1 diabetes this is particularly true of eating habits, while arterial risk is known to differ for the general population and people with Type 2 diabetes. Other care issues seem likely.

▷ Consideration

The group were aware of a systematic review designed to detect issues of relevance (rather than trials of interventions) and identified papers concerning differences in incidence, attitudes to complications, degree of response to education programmes, blood glucose control, religious fasting and feasting, and hospitalisation.

The group noted that cultural and genetic issues affected diabetes healthcare delivery in the areas of:

- patient education and self-care
- nutritional advice
- insulin therapy (including religious feasts and fasts)
- arterial risk
- blood pressure management
- hospitalisation.

In some areas there was overlap with social/deprivation issues. The group's recommendations address cultural/religious issues in the appropriate sections of this guideline, emphasising the primacy of the individual in this regard.

RECOMMENDATION

R37   Each adult with Type 1 diabetes should be managed as an individual, rather than as   D
       a member of any cultural, economic or health-affected group. Attention should be
       paid to the recommendations given elsewhere in this guideline with respect to the
       cultural preferences of individual adults with Type 1 diabetes.

7 | Blood glucose control and insulin therapy

7.1   Clinical monitoring of blood glucose

▷   Rationale

Type 1 diabetes is for most of the time asymptomatic once effective therapy is instituted. However, it is generally understood that there is a relationship between blood glucose control and the late complications of the condition. Together these observations suggest that some means of monitoring blood glucose control should help healthcare professionals advise people with diabetes to best effect on insulin doses, regimens and associated lifestyle issues.

▷   Evidence statements

Glycated haemoglobin testing

A Diabetes UK consensus statement recommended that only HbA_{1c} should be used in the monitoring of blood glucose control. Other studies reported within a systematic review[89] have shown discrepancies in the classification of patients between HbA_{1c} and HbA_1 assays (**IV**).

Two studies in a systematic review[89] showed high inter-individual variability for GHb assays in non-diabetic and in diabetic subjects with stable or variable control. One of these studies suggested an association between clinical control and sampling interval (**IIa**).

The same systematic review[89] reported on randomised controlled trial evidence supporting the use of GHb measurements, in particular results cited from the DCCT demonstrated the usefulness of these assays in contributing to improved long-term blood glucose control and a reduction in morbidity (**Ia**).

A Danish systematic review[108] reported that HbA_{1c} values allowed clinicians to identify patients with poor glycaemic control, concluding that GHb is the most clinically appropriate test of long-term glycaemia and should be used in routine management of Type 1 diabetes (**Ia**).

Frequency of monitoring

The optimal frequency of testing has not been established.

One study within a systematic review[89] recommended that no more than six GHb assays were necessary in a given year (**IV**).

ADA recommendations[76] advise GHb measurements are performed in accordance with clinical judgements. ADA consensus recommends GHb testing at least twice a year in patients with stable glycaemic control who are meeting treatment goals. Testing should be more frequent (quarterly) in patients whose therapy has changed or who are not meeting glycaemic control targets (**IV**).

Fructosamine testing

There are discrepancies in the evidence surrounding the use of fructosamine testing.

One study within a systematic review[89] reported fructosamine testing as able to detect shorter or more recent fluctuations in blood glucose compared to GHb. Fructosamine testing does not have the problems of standardisation associated with GHb, thus results are comparable between laboratories (**IIa**).

Two studies within a systematic review[89] described a high correlation between fructosamine and HbA_{1c}, however later studies debated this claim. One study suggested that although fructosamine correlates with HbA_{1c}, the value of HbA_{1c} in an individual cannot routinely be inferred with reliability from the level of fructosamine (**IIa**).

Two studies contained within a systematic review,[89] in patients with renal failure and elderly Type 2 diabetes patients with liver cirrhosis and nephrotic syndrome, suggest the influence of chronic conditions rather than metabolic control on fructosamine levels is the source of unreliability in test result. The systematic review concludes that more evidence is needed to resolve these issues (**IV**).

One correlation study within a review[89] showed no significant correlation between HbA_{1c} and fructosamine results over a six month follow-up (**III**).

Frequency of monitoring

ADA recommendations[76] state that assays of glycated serum protein would have to be performed on a monthly basis to gather the same information as measured in GHb three to four times per year (**IV**).

A systematic review[89] urges caution in using fructosamine testing, in light of the fact that fructosamine values can be improved by increased concordance a week or two before testing (**IV**).

Another study found that fasting blood glucose level (FBG) and serum fructosamine are not as useful as HbA_{1c} for monitoring diabetic control, but are additional extras for assessing control over short and long periods[89] (**IIa**).

Continuous glucose monitoring systems

Three observational studies[109–111] compared continuous glucose monitoring systems (CGMS) with SMBG. Studies demonstrated good correlation of CGMS with plasma and capillary measures of blood glucose over a range of blood glucose values. Error grid analysis showed the majority of readings fell within a clinically acceptable margin of error across all studies (**III**).

One study[111] reported acceptable level of comfort with CGMS. However, none of these studies address viable outcomes of glycaemic control or long-term use. Study methodology is not clearly reported (**III**).

Near patient testing

In this guideline, 'near patient testing' is defined as a biochemical or other test at or near (in time and place) the clinical consultation, such that the result is available at the consultation.

One controlled trial within a systematic review[112] demonstrated that near patient testing led to an increase in management changes for patients with poor glucose control. Near patient testing for HbA$_{1c}$ improved the process of care of patients (IIa).

In the same review,[112] questionnaires recording patient satisfaction of near patient testing concluded that the introduction of near patient testing for HbA$_{1c}$ improves the likelihood of monitoring and discussion of glycaemic control at patient visits. Patients reported that this was important to them and resulted in greater satisfaction with the test information provided (III).

Within the health technology assessment,[112] a retrospective cohort study showed that, after allowing for confounding factors, mean HbA$_{1c}$ level was lower following near patient testing and the immediate availability of results. In order to precisely quantify the effect of the testing system on HbA$_{1c}$ level, further, prospective studies are required (IIa).

A systematic review[89] reported four studies on the effectiveness of benchtop analysers compared with traditional laboratory methods. Two studies showed comparable results between the two techniques when operated by non-medical personnel. One study found that the benchtop analyser, although reliable, tended to slightly underestimate HbA$_{1c}$, compared with high performance liquid chromatography (HPLC) (IIa).

▷ Health economic evidence

An HTA report[112] produced cost estimates for near patient testing conducted by a laboratory or nurse against conventional testing. However, little data was available on the effects of near patient testing on clinical or quality of life outcomes. For health economics to provide guidance in this area, the long-term effects of different types of clinical monitoring on glycaemic control and subsequent complications must be known.

A recent HTA report[89] recommended further research into the cost-effectiveness of near patient testing for diabetes, FBG and fructosamine testing. No other paper in the health economics searches specifically addressed the issue of clinical monitoring.

▷ Consideration

The group endorsed the utility of having a frame of reference against which people with diabetes and the professionals advising them could assess risk and risk threshold for micro- and macro-vascular disease in terms of blood glucose control. This was a core component of intensification of therapy in studies showing improved long-term outcomes. HbA$_{1c}$ is the only measure for which quantitative information linking glucose control to complications is available, and then only when standardised to the assay used in the DCCT study. Near patient testing was felt to be a core component of making optimal and relevant use of HbA$_{1c}$ results. Continuous glucose monitoring systems were considered to not yet have established their usefulness beyond problem-solving in the occasional person with recurrent blood glucose control problems at the same time of day.

RECOMMENDATIONS

R38   Clinical monitoring of blood glucose levels by high precision DCCT-aligned methods   D
of haemoglobin A_{1c} (HbA_{1c}) should be performed every two to six months depending on:

- achieved level of blood glucose control
- stability of blood glucose control
- change in insulin dose or regimen.

R39   Site-of-care measurement, or measurement before clinical consultation, should be   D
provided.

R40 HbA_{1c} results should be communicated to the person with Type 1 diabetes after each   D
measurement. The term 'A1c' can be used for simplicity.

R41   Total glycated haemoglobin (GHb) estimation, or assessment of glucose profiles, should   A
be used where haemoglobinopathy or haemoglobin turnover invalidate HbA_{1c}
measurement.

R42   Fructosamine should not be used as a routine substitute for HbA_{1c} estimation.   B

R43   Continuous glucose monitoring systems have a role in the assessment of glucose   B
profiles in adults with consistent glucose control problems on insulin therapy, notably:

- repeated hyper- or hypoglycaemia at the same time of day
- hypoglycaemia unawareness, unresponsive to conventional insulin dose adjustment.

7.2   Glucose control assessment levels

▷   Rationale

The DCCT, and a number of smaller studies which are potentially underpowered,[113] suggest that more intensive management of people with Type 1 diabetes (by themselves, with advice) reduces the rate of development of microvascular complications over a period of years. The primary metabolic improvement in the DCCT was lowering of blood glucose level, and this was the measure used in that study to drive the intensification of therapy. This suggests that using measures of blood glucose control in the routine management of therapy in people with Type 1 diabetes is well founded.

A question then arises as to what level of blood glucose control people with diabetes should choose to strive for. A closely related question is what level(s) of glucose control should be used in assessing the performance of diabetes services.

'Targets' have been criticised by some as not giving flexibility for individuals with particular problems (eg hypoglycaemia) to be content with higher HbA_{1c} levels, which allows some longer-term risk for a gain in current well-being. It is clearly useful to be able to identify those in whom newer and more expensive technologies could be tried in an attempt to reduce microvascular risk, and to distinguish them from those who already achieve safe (or safer) levels on their current therapy. People with diabetes need information on what blood glucose level they need to attain if they wish to minimise vascular risk.

▷ Evidence statements – guidelines

In 1989, the European NIDDM Policy Group (Type 2 diabetes) suggested HbA_1 was good <8.5%, acceptable 8.5–9.5%, poor >9.5% (equivalent to HbA_{1c} of <6.9, 6.9–7.7, >7.7%). No evidence for these limits was given, and it was not clear whether the intent was for micro- or macrovascular protection or both. However, the need to individualise by life expectancy was acknowledged[114] (**IV**).

In 1993, the above guidelines were revised to HbA_{1c} <6.5%, 6.5–7.5%, and >7.5%. The European IDDM Policy Group (Type 1 diabetes) (WHO, IDF, St Vincent) met concurrently and agreed these, but using the terminology 'good', 'borderline' and 'poor' to describe the groups. These pre-DCCT recommendations are not justified in the text[115] (**IV**). See Table 3, below, for how that guideline maps these assessment levels to self-monitored blood glucose equivalents.

Table 3 Blood glucose equivalents (self-monitored) of HbA_{1c} assessment levels, as given in the 1993 European IDDM Policy Group guideline		
HbA_{1c} (%)	Pre-prandial (mmol/l)	Post-prandial (mmol/l)
6.5	6.1	8.0
7.5	8.0	10.0

In 1998, the European Diabetes Policy Group revised its terminology to 'assessment levels', giving advice on how to use assessment levels to set targets for individuals. These were, for HbA_{1c}: adequate 6.2–7.5%, inadequate >7.5%. However the relation of this 7.5% to glucose levels was then revised to equivalent to a self-monitored pre-prandial level of 6.5 mmol/l and post-prandial 9.0 mmol/l. These post-DCCT recommendations are not justified in the text[115] (**III**).

The NICE (inherited) Type 2 diabetes guideline on glucose control reads (**NICE**):

Evidence: narrative

The UKPDS showed that the reduction over a median of 10 years in HbA_{1c} from 7.9 to 7.0% using sulphonylureas or insulin provided much of the benefit that could be expected from that degree of improved glycaemic control. However it also illustrated the difficulties in being able to reach this level (7.0%) in a substantial proportion of people. Thus providing only one target is likely to encounter a significant number of people who 'fail' to meet that target. Similarly for some individuals an even lower target is desirable as they may have additional risk factors which necessitates even tighter blood glucose control. The UKPDS also suggested that there were no thresholds for cessation of benefit and that the lower the level of mean HbA_{1c} the better.

Working group commentary

The Working group tried to reflect these issues when deciding upon a target HbA_{1c}. They concluded that a range was the best option, recognising the difficulty in achieving a low target whilst recognising the importance of trying to achieve as near normal an HbA_{1c} level as possible, and in particular recognising that additional risk factors made the lower limit even more important for many individuals. While no study suggests clear thresholds, the group noted on the basis of the epidemiological evidence in the DCCT (Type 1 diabetes) and UKPDS that microvascular risk was low once average HbA_{1c} was around 7.0–8.0% while arterial risk continued to fall down to 6.0 to 7.0% (DCCT standardised).

Thus the target for each individual should be set which fully takes into account: their assessed risk factors, including: age, BMI, blood pressure and lipid status, side effects of therapy, other individual factors, patient choice.[382]

The NICE Type 2 diabetes guidelines therefore recommended 6.5% to 7.5% as ideal targets, individualised by balance of macrovascular (tend to 6.5%) and microvascular (7.5%) risk (**NICE**).

The ADA has republished its recommendations yearly.[76] These choose a 'glycaemic goal' of HbA_{1c} <7.0% for adults (type of diabetes not specified), equating this to pre-prandial <7.2 mmol/l and peak post-prandial <10.0 mmol/l. However, a table in the same paper suggests that an HbA_{1c} of 7.0% equates to mean self-monitored plasma glucose of 9.5 mmol/l[116] (**IV**).

However in the same issue (January 2003),[76] the ADA notes in a chapter on 'Implications of the DCCT' that the level of glucose control to be sought under ideal circumstances is an HbA_{1c} of around 7.2% (average glucose 8.6 mmol/l). This argument is based on that achieved in the DCCT, and is thus not theoretically justified (**IV**).

The microvascular risk threshold is what determines the diagnostic threshold for diabetes. In theory, oral glucose tolerance test (OGTT) findings should give some guidance as to this threshold. Unfortunately these are mainly based on non-physiological glucose load findings, and set a top limit of risk for 2h post-prandial levels. Fasting levels have been set as a microvascular threshold of 7.0 mmol/l (based on epidemiological equivalence with 2h OGTT levels), which would map to a DCCT-harmonised HbA_{1c} of about 7.7% (**IV**).

▷   Evidence statements

Simple direct findings indicating the microvascular risk level for people with Type 1 diabetes are not available.

The DCCT data has never been satisfactorily analysed with a view to answering this question. A graph in the original main paper[117] suggests a curvilinear relationship between control and complications, giving the conclusion that lower is always better (ignoring the hypoglycaemia issue for this purpose), down at least to the levels measured in the study (5.5%). This conclusion is called into question because (**IIa**):

- it is based on study averages, and even people at lower levels over nine years may have been at high levels at times
- it takes no account of pre-trial levels
- incident retinopathy is counted only in a forward (worsening) direction, which makes no allowance for false negative retinopathy at baseline
- worsening retinopathy is known to occur in the first two years after improvement of blood glucose control, and this is not discounted.

Further analysis was published in 1995.[118] Unfortunately, this is mostly in the form of a series of fitted curves without the data on which they are based. Curves of risk *vs* time suggest that retinopathy progression in the intensively managed group did not increase with time with a mean HbA_{1c} of 8.0%, and increased little at this level in the conventionally managed group with time (**IIa**).

Reanalysis of the published DCCT curve[118] suggests no worsening of retinopathy rates from normal levels until HbA_{1c} >8.0%; the 'low' rates (2% per 100 patient years) below that may be artefact for the reasons given above. The UKPDS (epidemiological analysis, Type 2 diabetes, microvascular disease) suffers much the same problems.[119] A similar level is found for retinopathy of 2% per 100 patient years at an HbA_{1c} of 7.5% and of 1% per 100 patient years at a level of 6.5% (III).

One study (1989)[120] studied HbA_1 and retinopathy incidence long term in Belfast. While some clear relationships were established the data showing no proliferative retinopathy below an HbA_1 of 10.0% (HbA_{1c} 8.5%) are compromised by very small numbers, and only interquartile ranges are given for non-proliferative retinopathy (III).

Neither the Oslo nor Stockholm studies of control and complications in Type 1 diabetes[121] give useful data on targets and thresholds, beyond showing that people with lower levels on average do better (III).

A non-randomised controlled study[122] looked prospectively at glycated Hb and micro-albuminuria risk in people with Type 1 diabetes attending their clinic. Their data did suggest a threshold effect (small and unchanging incidence below threshold, sharp rise above), at 7.9–8.5% HbA_{1c} (the authors chose to centre on 8.1%) (IIa).

A non-randomised controlled study[123] looked at how glycated Hb measurement related to OGTT results, performing a meta-analysis on 18 studies. Unfortunately most of these were published before any kind of GHb standardisation, rendering the results uninterpretable (IIa).

A further cohort study[124] looked in more detail at GHb, fasting and 2h glucose as diagnostic methods (and thus mainly Type 2 diabetes), using retinopathy and nephropathy as outcome measures. It may be noted that the Wisconsin data suggested that the microvascular/glucose control relationships were the same in Type 1 and Type 2 diabetes. The data presentations are strongly reminiscent of previous work,[122] with low and unchanging incidence of microvascular disease up to an inflection point, then sharply rising rates. The thresholds for fasting glucose appear to be somewhere above 6.8 mmol/l (consistent with older OGTT data), and HbA_{1c} somewhere above 7.4% (and below 9.1%) (IIa).

Glucose equivalents

Two non-randomised controlled studies[116,125] report the relationship between HbA_{1c} and self-monitored pre- and post-prandial glucose levels. The reports are consistent and can be related to DCCT-harmonised assays. It must be noted that these studies used pre-determined, self-monitored profiles taken from memory meters, and cannot easily be translated into patient-selected estimations, or only pre-prandial monitoring. They also omit the effects of night-time glucose profiles between bedtime and pre-breakfast readings. These data give the most robust evidence of the relationship between HbA_{1c} and the toxic glucose concentrations which actually cause the microvascular damage (IIa).

▷ Consideration

There must be a threshold for glucose control and the development of microvascular complications, or non-diabetic people would get complications. Indeed, this threshold must be well above the normal range as people with impaired glucose tolerance (IGT) do not (by definition) get microvascular complications. As people with IGT have HbA_{1c} levels of up to 7.0%, this by itself sets a lower limit of microvascular risk.

The microvascular thresholds of HbA_{1c} 7.5% set around 10 years ago have stood the test of all data published since. If anything the DCCT, Krolewski and McCance data suggest a figure closer to 8.0%.

Recommendations from the ADA (7.0%) and American College of Endocrinologists (6.5%) are not specific to type of diabetes; data does suggest macrovascular protection is gained by lowering blood glucose levels into the normal range, and the NICE (inherited) guidelines for Type 2 diabetes go for HbA_{1c} 6.5% in these higher arterial risk individuals.

Some people with Type 1 diabetes are at higher arterial risk, notably those with developing nephropathy. This can be identified by increased albumin excretion rate. The presence of features of the metabolic syndrome will also predict higher arterial risk. It may be appropriate to consider tighter targets for glucose control (if feasible) in people in these categories.

However, these levels are better considered as *assessment levels*, to be used in setting realistic targets for the individual. Major diabetes services in Europe currently only get about 20% of people with Type 1 diabetes into the sub-7.5% bracket. UK composite data (UKDIABS) shows some services doing better, but this may only represent non-standardised GHb estimation.

That current technologies of diabetes care markedly limited the proportion of people on insulin who were able to manage themselves to ideal levels was not seen as a bar to setting such assessment levels. It was noted that arterial risk would be likely to have a different relationship in this regard from microvascular risk, and that for the former there was little direct information available for people with Type 1 diabetes, but that the understandings gained in Type 2 diabetes and people without diabetes gave strong guidance in this respect. It was felt that as the assessment of the evidence available pointed to target definition in the same range as other published guidelines, and in particular the NICE inherited guidelines for Type 2 diabetes, there was practical utility for practice of care in having matching recommendations. Lastly the problem of hypoglycaemia in limiting was what achievable in any individual should be addressed within any recommendations, to assuage inappropriate attempts to achieve tight control and counter impressions of failure if targets are not attained.

RECOMMENDATIONS

R44   Adults with Type 1 diabetes should be advised that maintaining a DCCT-harmonised   **B**
        HbA_{1c} below 7.5% is likely to minimise their risk of developing diabetic eye, kidney
        or nerve damage in the longer term.

R45   Adults with Type 1 diabetes who want to achieve an HbA_{1c} down to, or towards,   **D**
        7.5% should be given all appropriate support in their efforts to do so.

R46   Where there is evidence of increased arterial risk (identified by a raised albumin   **NICE**
        excretion rate, features of the metabolic syndrome, or other arterial risk factors) people
        with Type 1 diabetes should be advised that approaching lower HbA_{1c} levels (for
        example 6.5% or lower) may be of benefit to them. Support should be given to
        approaching this target if so wished.

R47   Where target HbA_{1c} levels are not reached in the individual, adults with Type 1 diabetes   **B**
should be advised that any improvement is beneficial in the medium and long term,
and that greater improvements towards the target level lead to greater absolute gains.

R48   Undetected hypoglycaemia and an attendant risk of unexpected disabling hypoglycaemia   **D**
or of hypoglycaemia unawareness should be suspected in adults with Type 1 diabetes who
have:

- lower HbA_{1c} levels, in particular levels in or approaching the normal reference range
  (DCCT harmonised <6.1%)
- HbA_{1c} levels lower than expected from self-monitoring results.

R49   Where experience or risk of hypoglycaemia is significant to an individual, or the effort   **D**
needed to achieve target levels severely curtails other quality of life despite optimal use
of current diabetes technologies, tighter blood glucose control should not be pursued
without balanced discussion of the advantages and disadvantages.

*Note: A new chemical standard for HbA_{1c} has been developed by the International Federation of
Clinical Chemistry (IFCC). This reads lower by around 2.0% (units), and will be the basis of
primary calibration of instruments from 2004 onwards. However, this does not preclude the use of
DCCT-harmonised levels, and views from patient organisations and professional bodies at a recent
Department of Health meeting (July 2003) are that all HbA_{1c} reports should be DCCT aligned,
pending some internationally concerted policy change.*

7.3   Insulin regimens

▷   Rationale

Type 1 diabetes is an insulin deficiency disease. Physiological insulin delivery is regulated on a
minute-to-minute basis, while therapeutic insulin is given a small number of times a day.
Furthermore subcutaneous depot insulin preparations have, until recently, not come close to
providing the physiological plasma insulin profiles occurring at mealtimes or in the inter-
prandial basal state. A number of preparations of mealtime and extended-acting insulins are
available, and combining these to suit individual needs, while taking account of preferences for
numbers of injections, gives a variety of possible insulin regimens of differing characteristics.

While insulin deficiency is the hallmark of Type 1 diabetes, a few people retain some insulin
secretion for a short time (and might therefore benefit from insulin secretagogues). Some
glucose-lowering drugs work on gut absorption of nutrients or on the insulin effector tissues,
and might therefore be expected to be of benefit in some individuals even when completely
insulin deficient and managed on insulin replacement therapy.

▷   Evidence statements

Insulin and insulin analogues

Insulin with the molecular structure of human and animal insulins is currently available.
Evidence from the majority of studies[126–8] reports no significant differences in hypoglycaemic
episodes and glycaemic control between the insulin of human and animal chemical
structures (**Ia**).

Conventional two-dose insulin regimens may result in a high frequency of nocturnal hypoglycaemia. Intensified three-dose insulin regimens improve glycaemic control, but often do not improve morning blood glucose[129] (**Ia**).

Continuous subcutaneous insulin infusion (CSII) improves nocturnal and morning glycaemic control compared with multiple daily injection (MDI) regimens. With multiple injection regimens the morning injection must not be delayed. Total and bolus insulin doses required are lower with CSII compared with MDI[130] (**Ib**).

Mortality from acute metabolic causes (ketoacidosis) was reported as significantly increased with intensified treatment; odds ratio 7.20 (pumps) 1.13 (multiple daily injection).[129] The pump data is however based on early pump technologies (**Ia**).

Similar glycaemic control results from either lente or isophane (NPH) insulin when used as basal insulin for multiple injection regimens together with a short-acting insulin preparation before meals[131] (**Ib**).

On the balance of effectiveness and cost-effectiveness evidence, insulin glargine, which has a peakless action profile, is also recommended as a long-acting preparation for people with Type 1 diabetes;[132] some studies in this review show significantly lower fasting blood glucose with insulin glargine than isophane (NPH) insulin and others suggest that people on insulin glargine may experience fewer hypoglycaemic events than people receiving once-daily isophane (NPH) insulin[132] (**NICE**).

Evidence from a large multicentred study suggests that people commonly inject insulin closer to mealtime than the recommended 30 minutes. Due to slow absorption and delayed action, the use of unmodified ('soluble') human insulin as pre-meal dose results in high and variable post-breakfast blood glucose concentrations, which together with the incidence of later hypoglycaemia suggests that this regimen does not give satisfactory post-prandial blood glucose control in many patients[133] (**Ib**).

Rapid acting insulin analogues allow injection closer to mealtimes due to their pharmacokinetic profile[134–6] (**Ib**).

A meta-analysis[137] and several open-label trials[133,138–145] show that insulin lispro is more effective than unmodified ('soluble') human insulin in improving post-prandial glucose control, without an increase in the rate of hypoglycaemic episodes (**Ia**).

Two studies[146–7] show reduced frequency of nocturnal hypoglycaemia[148] with insulin lispro compared to unmodified ('soluble') human insulin (**Ib**).

Two studies[148–9] show reduced frequency of severe hypoglycaemia with insulin lispro compared to unmodified ('soluble') human insulin (**Ia**).

Patients perceive an improvement in their well-being and quality of life with rapid-acting insulin analogues due to flexibility of injection times and less frequent hypoglycaemic reactions[128,141,146] (**Ib**).

The effects of insulin lispro on HbA_{1c} levels (overall glycaemic control) have not been firmly established.[133,137,149] The long-term safety profile is as yet unknown (**Ia**).

Two multicentre randomised studies[149–50] and one RCT[135] showed insulin aspart to improve post-prandial glucose control more effectively than unmodified ('soluble') human insulin, without an increase in the rate of hypoglycaemic episodes. Fewer major hypoglycaemic episodes were observed (**Ia**).

A before-and-after study has shown that a lower dose of mealtime insulin can be taken along with an increase in basal dose, with no increase in hypoglycaemic episodes when insulin lispro is used as a replacement for human insulin as mealtime injection therapy[142] (**IIb**).

Two randomised trials have shown that it is possible to replace mealtime unmodified ('soluble') human insulin with insulin lispro or insulin aspart without detriment to glycaemic control if care is taken to replace basal insulin delivery more physiologically[151–2] (**Ib**).

A multi-arm randomised trial found that adding a few units of isophane (NPH) insulin to insulin lispro at each meal, in combination with bedtime NPH insulin improves blood glucose concentrations compared to an unmodified ('soluble') human insulin regimen in a multidose regimen[136] (**Ib**).

Splitting the evening administration of insulin to short-acting insulin at dinner and isophane (NPH) insulin at bedtime has a number of advantages over mixed administration of short-acting insulin and isophane (NPH) at dinner. Compared with the mixed mealtime regimen, the evening split regimen reduced by more than 60% the risk of nocturnal hypoglycaemia;[153–4] improved long-term control of blood glucose levels, decreased variability of blood glucose levels in fasting state and led to improvement in preserved hormonal, symptom and cognitive function responses to hypoglycaemia (**Ib**).

When basal insulin replacement is by either continuous subcutaneous insulin infusion (CSII) or multiple daily administrations of isophane (NPH) insulin, the long term administration of lispro at mealtime reduces HbA_{1c};[130] however, compared with multiple daily injections, patients using continuous subcutaneous administration of insulin (mainly those using older systems) have been at a significantly higher risk of ketoacidosis (**Ib**).

Frequency of hypoglycaemic reactions was found to be similar on patient-mixed and premixed insulins.[143,155] One randomised controlled trial showed premixed preparations of insulin analogues to be well suited for those who wish to limit the number of daily injections;[155] 83% of people expressed a preference for premixed insulins throughout the trial (**Ib**).

Few studies have addressed the needs of people with diabetes with suboptimal glucose control, and none of suitable design from the evidence hierarchy were found for review.

In a group of people with Type 1 diabetes with poor glucose control, the introduction of more intensive insulin regimens may lead to high loss to follow-up.[156]

Poor outcome appears to be due to the people refusing the constraints of multiple daily injections, effective blood glucose self-monitoring and regular clinic visits at short time intervals. It was suggested that people should be given clear and concise information on treatment goals and the ways in which these goals are to be attained as well as an explanation of the advantages and disadvantages (**IV**).

Few studies addressed the needs of people newly diagnosed with diabetes and none of suitable design from the evidence hierarchy were found for review.

Acarbose and insulin combination therapy

Four randomised controlled trials, two large parallel groups,[157–8] and two small crossover designs[159–60] were identified that examined the use of acarbose in conjunction with insulin therapy compared to insulin and placebo in each case, in people with Type 1 diabetes. A multicentred study[157] with variable doses titrated up to 300 mg three times a day for 24 weeks, found a significant reduction in HbA$_{1c}$ levels with acarbose compared to placebo, and decreases in fasting and post-prandial glucose levels to two hours. There were no differences between groups for daily insulin dose or hypoglycaemic events, although adverse events of abdominal pain, diarrhoea and flatulence were more common with acarbose. This led to more frequent treatment discontinuation in the acarbose group than the placebo group. A similar Italian trial[158] with up to 100 mg acarbose three times daily for 24 weeks found no difference in HbA$_{1c}$ levels, daily insulin dose, fasting glycaemia and total cholesterol. However, a significant decrease was found in two-hour post-prandial plasma glucose level, and HDL cholesterol levels were lower in people on acarbose than placebo. Again minor adverse events were more common in the acarbose group, but hypoglycaemic episodes were similar in both groups. Although care was taken not to alter baseline insulin doses, this could be adjusted if glucose levels exceeded 11.1 mmol/l or reduced with hypoglycaemic episodes (**Ib**).

The two crossover trials with 100 mg acarbose three times a day over relatively short time periods did not assess requirement for wash out periods (although analysis in one found no effect of treatment order) and did not account for study withdrawals. One study found a benefit in terms of HbA$_{1c}$ with acarbose,[160] while the other found no significant differences between groups.[159] Potential methodological limitations of these trials would not permit them to be used as an evidence base to inform recommendations in this area (**Ib**).

Sulfonylurea and insulin combination therapy

Two small randomised controlled trials investigated the use of glibenclamide (called 'glyburide' as the trials were conducted in the USA) in the therapy for Type 1 diabetics. A study using 5 mg glyburide (orally) for 12 weeks compared to placebo after a 12-week open-label insulin stabilisation run-in period[161] found fasting blood glucose declined significantly at 12 weeks from baseline, although no comparison was made between groups. No differences were found in daily insulin dose or glycated haemoglobin levels at any stage of the study. A randomised study without comparison between groups at baseline with 5 mg glyburide daily for 24 weeks compared to placebo[162] found no differences in plasma C-peptide levels between groups, nor difference in plasma glucose concentrations at any time point. Although HbA$_{1c}$ levels were reported to have changed more from baseline in the glyburide treated group at six weeks, potential methodological limitations of these trials would not permit them to be used as an evidence base to inform recommendations in this area (**Ib**).

Comparison of 15 mg of glibenclamide daily with placebo in addition to insulin therapy in a small sample of people with Type 1 diabetes in a randomised double-blind crossover study[163] found mean blood glucose level, HbA$_{1c}$ and blood glucose variability to be significantly lower with the intervention among people who retained endogenous insulin production. No such differences were found in a subgroup who were C-peptide negative. Although the study had a medium-term intervention period of three months, it did not provide analysis of the cohort as a whole for glibenclamide *vs* placebo and thus cannot be used for recommendations given the small sample sizes of the subgroups, and the inherent difficulties of extrapolating such findings to a wider population (**Ib**).

A reduced insulin requirement at 18 months was found in patients given 80 mg gliclazide twice a day compared to placebo in a small sample in a long-term study.[164] Although glycated haemoglobin both fasting and one hour post-breakfast were found to be very similar in both groups, the gliclazide group had C-peptide levels significantly higher than people on placebo for the same test times of the day, at six-monthly assessment points to 18 months. This study only applies to people with retained endogenous insulin secretion, and thus not the overwhelming majority of people with Type 1 diabetes (**Ib**).

Metformin

A medium-sized randomised controlled study found that the addition of metformin to an insulin regimen provided by CSII was able to reduce the total IR required by the person with Type 1 diabetes (including reduced basal therapy) as compared to placebo over a period of six months. This was achieved without significant change to HbA_{1c} or increased incidence of hypoglycaemia (**Ib**).

▷ Health economic evidence

The health economic searches produced no studies giving guidance on appropriate insulin regimens for those newly-diagnosed with Type 1 diabetes or for the management and prevention of hypoglycaemia, with the exception of the NICE appraisal of insulin glargine.

The health economic searches found no published papers dealing with insulin glargine or NPH insulin. A recent NICE technology appraisal[132] recommended insulin glargine as a long-acting preparation for people with Type 1 diabetes alongside insulin NPH. The crucial issue for the cost-effectiveness of insulin glargine is the amount of utility associated with reducing the fear of hypoglycaemia.

Two cost-benefit studies were identified that considered the role of insulin lispro.[342,380] Neither paper was based in the UK (Canada, Australia), and both suggest that the willingness to pay for insulin lispro will outweigh its additional cost. The cost-effectiveness of lispro is unclear and is likely to be most favourable amongst those who require increased flexibility in setting mealtimes, or those for whom mealtimes are often unpredictable.

The issue of the cost-effectiveness of intensive insulin therapy is complicated by a shortage of unconfounded data. The DCCT showed that a series of interventions including intensive insulin therapy reduces the rate of diabetic complications and increases life expectancy amongst an unrepresentative sample of adults and adolescents with Type 1 diabetes. Because of the complexity of this intervention, health economic analysis of the DCCT data has typically assumed that these reductions are primarily due to intensive insulin regimens.

The health economic searches found three models designed to find the cost-effectiveness of intensive treatment,[343–4,381] of which two attempted to form QALYs. The health utility values in each of the studies are poor: in one study[343] non-preference-based values are used; in another[381] only a very small sample was used to find health utilities. Both studies considered only a small number of health states and both suggest that intensive therapy is cost-effective.

Two models analysed intensive treatment in cost-per-life-year terms, and differed in their results. One study[343] produced a cost-per-life-year figure of US$28,661 at 1994 prices, whilst another[344] found a figure several times larger. Neither study used UK costs. Note that as several diabetic complications will affect quality of life but will not significantly shorten life expectancy, the cost-per-QALY figure may be lower than the corresponding cost-per-life-year figure. Two cost analyses also suggest that the DCCT cost estimates may be overestimates.[345–6] Few inferences can be drawn because these studies are limited but it appears likely that intensive treatment, including intensive insulin regimens, will be cost-effective.

▷ Consideration

It was noted that Type 1 diabetes is a hormone deficiency disease. The problems faced by people with the condition (injections, hypoglycaemia, hyperglycaemia, consequences of capricious control, late complications) were noted to be solely a function of the poor state of insulin replacement therapy.

The group noted that the use of insulin injections in people with Type 1 diabetes is not RCT-based and never could be. It was also noted that, prior to the introduction of short- and long-acting insulin analogues, the use of insulin regimens based on a combination in various forms of unmodified (soluble) human insulin before meals and human isophane (NPH) insulin for basal supply had become widespread, and that, the analogues aside, there was no evidence to challenge that conventional practice. Long-acting analogues, or rather insulin glargine, are covered by NICE appraisal guidance, and this recommends their availability for use in people with Type 1 diabetes. Rapid-acting insulin analogues are supported by an evidence base for less hypoglycaemia at night and at some other times, reduced hyperglycaemic excursions after meals and small improvements in HbA_{1c}, suggesting that these too should have an increasing role in people with Type 1 diabetes.

The group was aware that the evidence for combining the advantages of rapid- and long-acting insulin analogues was evolving as the knowledge base to use these technologies improves. This combination would be particularly suitable to matching with active mealtime insulin dose adjustment (AMIDA, see dietary recommendations in 6.3). Some recent NICE technology appraisals provided a health economic basis for supporting this regimen, should appropriate improvements in HbA_{1c} be demonstrated. Accordingly the recommendations were drafted to allow choice of human or combined analogue regimens including from the time of diagnosis.

The group noted the potential usefulness of the new insulins in some special situations, including religious feasts and fasts, and shift work. A need to address insulin starters and people who wished for smaller numbers of injections was identified. A need to caution against using newer, more expensive insulins in people with control problems without proper assessment of underlying causes was felt appropriate. The NICE appraisal of insulin pumps (effectively an insulin regimen rather than a device) was noted, and no elaboration felt to be needed on that.

The group found the evidence for the general recommendation of any glucose-lowering drug in combination with insulin to be unconvincing. While there may be a small gain in overall glucose control evidenced inconsistently in the acarbose studies, the size of this gain, the prevalence of intolerance, and the suggestion of increased hypoglycaemia, together were taken as indicating that no recommendation for the general use of this drug in this context could be made.

The use of metformin and insulin sensitisers in people with Type 1 diabetes and the metabolic syndrome has not been adequately investigated.

The group was aware of the concern that arterial complications in people with Type 1 diabetes were associated with features of the metabolic syndrome as seen in Type 2 diabetes, and that there was evidence of benefit in people with Type 2 diabetes for some drugs, notably metformin (UKPDS study) and PPAR-γ agonists (see NICE guidance). While not endorsing the general use of such drugs in people with Type 1 diabetes and features of the metabolic syndrome (see section 8.2, 'Arterial disease management'), the group noted that further investigation might support the high *a priori* likelihood of benefit in this high-risk situation.

RECOMMENDATIONS

R50	Adults with Type 1 diabetes should have access to the types (preparation and species) of insulin they find allow them optimal well-being.	A
R51	Cultural preferences need to be discussed and respected in agreeing the insulin regimen for a person with Type 1 diabetes.	D
R52	Multiple insulin injection regimens, in adults who prefer them, should be used as part of an integrated package of which education, food and skills training should be integral parts.	A
R53	Appropriate self-monitoring and education should be used as part of an integrated package to help achieve optimal diabetes outcomes.	D
R54	Mealtime insulin injections should be provided by injection of unmodified ('soluble') insulin or rapid-acting insulin analogues before main meals.	D
R55	Rapid-acting insulin analogues should be used as an alternative to mealtime unmodified insulin: • where nocturnal or late inter-prandial hypoglycaemia is a problem • in those in whom they allow equivalent blood glucose control without use of snacks between meals and this is needed or desired.	A
R56	Basal insulin supply (including nocturnal insulin supply) should be provided by the use of isophane (NPH) insulin or long-acting insulin analogues (insulin glargine). Isophane (NPH) insulin should be given at bedtime. If rapid-acting insulin analogues are given at mealtimes or the midday insulin dose is small or lacking, the need to give isophane (NPH) insulin twice daily (or more often) should be considered.	D
R57	Long-acting insulin analogues (insulin glargine) should be used when: • nocturnal hypoglycaemia is a problem on isophane (NPH) insulin • morning hyperglycaemia on isophane (NPH) insulin results in difficult daytime blood glucose control • rapid-acting insulin analogues are used for mealtime blood glucose control.	D
R58	Twice-daily insulin regimens should be used by those adults who consider number of daily injections an important issue in quality of life: • biphasic insulin preparations (pre-mixes) are often the preparations of choice in this circumstance	D

- biphasic rapid-acting insulin analogue pre-mixes may give an advantage to those prone to hypoglycaemia at night.

Such twice daily regimens may also help:
- those who find adherence to their agreed lunchtime insulin injection difficult
- adults with learning difficulties who may require assistance from others.

R59	Adults whose nutritional and physical activity patterns vary considerably from day-to-day, for vocational or recreational reasons, may need careful and detailed review of their self-monitoring and insulin injection regimen(s). This should include all the appropriate preparations (see R55–7) and consideration of unusual patterns and combinations.	D

R60	For adults undergoing periods of fasting or sleep following eating (such as during religious feasts and fasts or after night-shift work), a rapid-acting insulin analogue before the meal (provided the meal is not prolonged) should be considered.	D

R61 For adults with erratic and unpredictable blood glucose control (hyper- and hypoglycaemia at no consistent times), rather than a change in a previously optimised insulin regimen, the following should be considered: **D**
- resuspension of insulin and injection technique
- injection sites
- self-monitoring skills
- knowledge and self-management skills
- nature of lifestyle
- psychological and psychosocial difficulties
- possible organic causes such as gastroparesis.

R62 Continuous subcutaneous insulin infusion (insulin pump therapy) is recommended as an option for people with Type 1 diabetes provided that: **NICE**
- multiple-dose insulin therapy (including, where appropriate, the use of insulin glargine) has failed;* and
- those receiving the treatment have the commitment and competence to use the therapy effectively.

R63 Partial insulin replacement to achieve blood glucose control targets (basal insulin only, or just some mealtime insulin) should be considered for adults starting insulin therapy, until such time as islet B-cell deficiency progresses further. **D**

R64 Clear guidelines and protocols ('sick day rules') should be given to all adults with Type 1 diabetes to assist them in adjusting insulin doses appropriately during intercurrent illness. **D**

R65 Oral glucose-lowering drugs should generally not be used in the management of adults with Type 1 diabetes. **D**

---

* People for whom multiple-dose therapy has failed are considered to be those for whom it has been impossible to maintain an HbA_{1c} level no greater than 7.5% (or 6.5% in the presence of microalbuminuria or adverse features of the metabolic syndrome) without disabling hypoglycaemia occurring, despite a high level of self-care of their diabetes. 'Disabling hypoglycaemia', for the purpose of this guidance, means the repeated and unpredicted occurrence of hypoglycaemia requiring third-party assistance that results in continuing anxiety about recurrence and is associated with significant adverse effect on quality of life.

7.4   Insulin delivery

▷   Rationale

As a large protein, insulin cannot be taken orally (it is digested) and is only absorbed across mucous membranes (of the nose or inside cheeks for example) very poorly. As a result, it generally has to be injected or infused into the subcutaneous fat. Self-use of injection devices is not something most people adopt happily by choice, and since the late 1970s various solutions to making this easier and more satisfactory have been developed.

▷   Evidence statements

NICE guidance[165] concluded that, compared to optimised MDI therapy, CSII results in a modest but worthwhile improvement in GHb and quality of life (by allowing greater flexibility of lifestyle), and reduction of other problems such as hypoglycaemia and rising blood glucose levels at the end of the night. In routine practice, patients who go on to pumps are carefully selected, and to a large degree self-selected. Overall, insulin pumps appear to be a useful advance for patients having particular problems, rather than a dramatic breakthrough in therapy, and would probably be used only in a small percentage of patients (**NICE**).

There is a paucity of trials of sufficient sample size in comparing insulin injection pens to other forms of insulin delivery.

One randomised trial[166] of medium sample size compared a multiple injection regimen from a pen injector with conventional treatment with twice-daily syringe injection. No significant differences were seen in GHb values, blood glucose values or hypoglycaemic episodes. Patient satisfaction with pen injectors was high and most patients opted to continue on this delivery system following termination of the trial. However, this study has some methodological limitations (**Ib**).

One randomised crossover trial[167] compared two types of insulin regimen injected in the abdomen with the same regimen injected in the thigh. Regular insulin injections in the abdomen resulted in significantly lower post-prandial plasma glucose values, peak plasma glucose and increment in plasma glucose compared to time periods following injection in the thigh. Significantly higher serum free insulin values were also seen following abdominal injection of regular insulin, compared with injections administered at the thigh. No differences were recorded between injections at either site following injections containing both isophane (NPH) and unmodified ('soluble') insulin (**Ib**).

One prospective study[168] comparing the absorption of insulin injected superficially and deep subcutaneously at the fat-muscle boundary showed no significant difference between the two techniques. A sub-group of 10 participants showed no difference in overall serum free insulin or plasma glucose values following superficial and deep subcutaneous injection (**IIa**).

One study[169] reported benefits associated with injection through clothing, compared with conventional injection practice with skin preparation over a 20-week trial period. This study had some methodological limitations (**Ib**).

Outside of the recommendations made on continuous subcutaneous insulin infusion,[165] no studies were identified that specifically addressed the insulin delivery needs of people with Type 1 diabetes with poor blood glucose control.

▷ Health economic evidence

The health economic searches produced three published papers[347–9] considering the use of insulin pens. None of the three papers compare their benefits (patient satisfaction, or improved HbA_{1c}) against their costs.

▷ Consideration

Insulin injection pens were noted to be the overwhelming norm in the UK for insulin delivery for reasons of convenience, ease of teaching and portability. Some devices with particular design characteristics can be used by people with disabilities, where otherwise a third party would have to give injections. The desirability and often cost-effectiveness of this was noted. Injection into deep subcutaneous fat, and on the basis of many studies into the tissues of the abdominal wall for mealtime unmodified human insulin, are generally advised and logically based. However the needs and beliefs of individuals in giving their own insulin were felt to be of importance. Simple logic also leads to the conclusion that rotation of injection sites should be within one region rather than between regions. Group members (both clinicians and people with diabetes) expressed a widespread experience of repeated self-injection with the same needle without problems arising. The group considered the utility of recommending advice on cleanliness for those who choose to re-use needles, but noted the regulatory position from the Medicines and Healthcare Products Regulatory Agency (MHRA, formerly the Medical Devices Agency) in the bulletin DB2000(04). Consequently, the guideline cannot make such a recommendation. Other common sense issues included provision for sharps disposal, and check on the condition of injection sites annually or if blood glucose control problems worsen.

RECOMMENDATIONS

| R66 | Adults with Type 1 diabetes who inject insulin should have access to the insulin injection delivery device they find allows them optimal well-being, often using one or more types of insulin injection pen. | D |

| R67 | Adults with Type 1 diabetes who have special visual or psychological needs should be provided with injection devices or needle-free systems that they can use independently for accurate dosing. | D |

| R68 | Insulin injection should be made into the deep subcutaneous fat. To achieve this, needles of a length appropriate to the individual should be made available. | D |

| R69 | Adults with Type 1 diabetes should be informed that the abdominal wall is the therapeutic choice for mealtime insulin injections. | D |

| R70 | Adults with Type 1 diabetes should be informed that extended-acting suspension insulin (for example isophane (NPH) insulin) may give a longer profile of action when injected into the subcutaneous tissue of the thigh rather than the arm or abdominal wall. | D |

| R71 | Adults with Type 1 diabetes should be recommended to use one anatomical area for the injections given at the same time of day, but to move the precise injection site around in the whole of the available skin within that area. | D |

R72   Adults with Type 1 diabetes should be provided with suitable containers for the   D
       collection of used needles. Arrangements should be available for the suitable disposal
       of these containers.

R73   Injection site condition should be checked annually, and if new problems with blood   D
       glucose control occur.

7.5   Hypoglycaemia: prevention of hypoglycaemia, problems related to hypoglycaemia and management of symptomatic hypoglycaemia

▷ Rationale

Hypoglycaemia is, for most people using insulin therapy, an inevitable consequence of the erratic absorption of insulin from subcutaneous tissue after depot injection or infusion, coupled with absence of feedback to insulin need when changes in planned activity or eating occur once the injection has been given. Hypoglycaemia is usually unpleasant, often becomes a source of fear, and can be an embarrassment as well as a safety risk. Accordingly, while careful choice of insulin regimen (section 7.3) informed by self-monitoring (section 6.2) is important in ameliorating this problem, other preventative measures are of importance. A higher level of optimised management is needed when hypoglycaemia and its related problems do occur.

▷ Evidence statements

Management of hypoglycaemia

Canadian clinical practice guidelines[98] reported four studies supporting the use of 15 g glucose (monosaccharide) (orally) for the treatment of moderate hypoglycaemia. Two studies within the guidelines explored a 20 g oral glucose dose for recovery of blood glucose levels. Recovery was slower following treatment with milk and orange juice. The use of glucose gel also delivered slower recovery in the latter study and required swallowing to have a significant effect. A further study showed no support for buccal administration of glucose (**Ia**).

One study within the Canadian guidelines[98] reported on the special needs of people taking alpha-glycosidase inhibitors when treating hypoglycaemia, recommending the use of glucose (dextrose) tablets, or milk or honey if these are unavailable (**IV**).

Nocturnal hypoglycaemia

A bedtime snack may be needed to avoid nocturnal hypoglycaemia. Two studies from a systematic review[98] showed prepared cornstarch snack bars have some benefit in overnight reduction of hypoglycaemia, but the number of events were not significantly reduced (**Ia**).

Hypoglycaemia unawareness

Canadian clinical practice guidelines[98] report one paper on the link between incidence of prior hypoglycaemic episodes and worsening in the defect of the hormonal responses to hypoglycaemia, leading to a reduction in the self-detection of hypoglycaemia. Eight papers report the benefits of strict avoidance of hypoglycaemia in improving recognition of severe hypoglycaemia or the responses of counter-regulatory hormones (**Ia**).

Blood glucose awareness training

A randomised controlled study[170] compared blood glucose awareness training (BGAT) with no training on the increased hypoglycaemia after initiation of more intensive diabetes management. The counter-regulatory hormone epinephrine (adrenaline) response was not impaired following BGAT despite an increase in frequency of hypoglycaemia induced by intensive diabetes management. No difference was seen in awareness of the symptoms of hypoglycaemia following BGAT, compared with controls, although BGAT does lead to a better detection of low blood glucose levels in people starting intensive diabetes management (**Ib**).

An observational study[171] compared blood glucose sensitivity and prediction accuracy in inpatients before and after blood glucose awareness training, showed no additional effect on the improvement of HbA_{1c}. The decrease in HbA_{1c} was not however accompanied by a change in the accuracy of blood glucose estimation or sensitivity of recognition of low blood glucose levels (**IIa**).

Canadian clinical practice guidelines[98] cite five studies demonstrating a positive effect of BGAT on accurate detection and treatment of hypoglycaemia, and allowing reduced-awareness subjects to detect a greater percentage of low blood glucose levels. These BGAT programmes involve instruction in interpretation of physical symptoms and instruction on food, exercise, insulin dosage and action, and the impact of time of day and last blood glucose measurements on estimations of blood glucose (**Ia**).

Long-term complications of hypoglycaemia

Evidence on the impact of hypoglycaemia on cognitive function is not clear. Two prospective studies reported within the Canadian guidelines[98] did not find association between intensive diabetes management and cognitive function. However, six retrospective studies found subjects with recurrent hypoglycaemia performed more poorly in a range of intellectual tests (**IIa**).

Medical intervention of hypoglycaemia

Two randomised studies compared the use of glucagon and dextrose in the treatment of severe hypoglycaemia. One study[172] compared intramuscular administration of 1 mg glucagon with 50 ml 50% IV dextrose in people with hypoglycaemic coma. A second study[173] compared intravenous administration of 1 mg glucagon *vs* 50 ml 50% dextrose in people with hypo-glycaemic coma. Both studies showed a significantly slower recovery to a normal level of consciousness in the glucagon treated group (**Ib**).

Two glucagon-treated patients in each study (7% and 4% respectively) and two dextrose-treated patients in the second study (4%) required additional administration of 12.5 g IV dextrose following failing to recover consciousness after 15 minutes. In the first study average duration of hypoglycaemic coma was not different between the two treatment groups (**Ib**).

No correlation was seen between time taken to recovery of consciousness and initial plasma glucose concentration or duration of hypoglycaemia in either of the studies. Side effects were similar among the treatment groups (**Ib**).

These two small studies suggest that intravenous glucose gives a clinically non-significant advantage over intramuscular glucagon in time to recovery of consciousness in people with Type 1 diabetes in hypoglycaemic coma (**Ib**).

▷ Health economics evidence

No health economic evidence on the prevention or management of hypoglycaemia was identified in the literature review.

▷ Consideration

The group noted this was an area of considerable importance to people with Type 1 diabetes, but that prevention of hypoglycaemia was considered appropriately under insulin therapy recommendations, and secondarily under education and lifestyle issues. The group noted issues related to absorption and ingestion of free carbohydrate in people with decreased conscious level. They were concerned that recurrent hypoglycaemia was properly considered in a medical context, and not simply attributed to lifestyle problems secondary to insulin therapy.

Hypoglycaemia unawareness was also noted to be an important issue, and be partially reversible and capable of useful management, as now is nocturnal hypoglycaemia (it was noted that the recommendations on insulin therapy and clinical monitoring addressed other aspects of such management). No useful hard evidence was available for cognitive decline occurring in people with Type 1 diabetes, but the possibility of recurrent severe hypoglycaemia being a contributory factor was felt worth mentioning.

The group noted that the ease and safety of administration of glucagon compared to IV glucose (risk of extravasation) meant that in most situations it was the treatment of choice. While it was recognised that there were groups of people to whom the identified studies do not apply (starvation, alcohol toxic), and that these people would not be expected to respond well to glucagon, it was agreed that the best means of detecting this was by absence of a response to glucagon at 10 minutes. Safe follow-up management after either therapy should include oral carbohydrate and awareness of risk of relapse. Users of glucagon injections need appropriate education and training.

RECOMMENDATIONS

R74   Adults with Type 1 diabetes should be informed that any available glucose/sucrose   **A** containing fluid is suitable for the management of hypoglycaemic symptoms or signs in people who are able to swallow. Glucose containing tablets or gels are also suitable for those able to dissolve or disperse these in the mouth and swallow the products.

R75   When a more rapid-acting form of glucose is required, purer glucose-containing   **D** solutions should be given.

R76   Adults with decreased level of consciousness due to hypoglycaemia who are unable to   **D** take oral treatment safely should be:
- given intramuscular glucagon by a trained user (intravenous glucose may be used by professionals skilled in obtaining intravenous access)
- monitored for response at 10 minutes, and then given intravenous glucose if the level of consciousness is not improving significantly
- then given oral carbohydrate when it is safe to administer it, and placed under continued observation by a third party who has been warned of the risk of relapse.

R77   Adults with Type 1 diabetes should be informed that some hypoglycaemic episodes are   B
an inevitable consequence of insulin therapy in most people using any insulin regimen,
and that it is advisable that they should use a regimen that avoids or reduces the
frequency of hypoglycaemic episodes while maintaining as optimal a level of blood
glucose control as is feasible. Advice to assist in obtaining the best such balance from
any insulin regimen should be available to all adults with Type 1 diabetes. (see section 7.2,
'Insulin regimens' and 7.2, 'Insulin delivery').

R78   When hypoglycaemia becomes unusually problematic or of increased frequency,   D
review should be made of the following possibly contributory causes:

- inappropriate insulin regimens (incorrect dose distributions and insulin types)
- meal and activity patterns including alcohol
- injection technique and skills including insulin resuspension
- injection site problems
- possible organic causes including gastroparesis
- changes in insulin sensitivity (the latter including drugs affecting the renin-
angiotensin system and renal failure)
- psychological problems
- previous physical activity
- lack of appropriate knowledge and skills for self-management.

R79   Hypoglycaemia unawareness should be assumed to be secondary to undetected   D
periods of hypoglycaemia (<3.5 mmol/l, often for extended periods, commonly at
night) until these are excluded by appropriate monitoring techniques. If present, such
periods of hypoglycaemia should be ameliorated.

R80   Specific education on the detection and management of hypoglycaemia in adults with   D
problems of hypoglycaemia awareness should be offered.

R81   Nocturnal hypoglycaemia (symptomatic or detected on monitoring) should be   D
managed by:

- reviewing knowledge and self-management skills
- reviewing current insulin regimen and evening eating habits and previous physical
activity
- choosing an insulin type and regimen with less propensity to induce low glucose levels in
the night hours, such as:
  - isophane (NPH) insulin at bedtime
  - rapid-acting analogue with the evening meal
  - long-acting insulin analogues (insulin glargine)
  - insulin pump.

R82   Adults with Type 1 diabetes should be informed that late post-prandial hypoglycaemia   D
may be managed by appropriate inter-prandial snacks, or the use of rapid-acting insulin
analogues before meals.

R83   Where early cognitive decline occurs in adults on long-term insulin therapy, normal   D
investigations should be supplemented by consideration or investigation of possible
brain damage due to overt or covert hypoglycaemia, and the need to ameliorate this.

8 | Arterial risk control

8.1   Identification of arterial risk

▷   Rationale

People with Type 1 diabetes are generally recognised to be at greatly increased risk of arterial disease (CVD) in middle age. While the literature on arterial risk factors and markers in the general population is large, it would not appear to follow that the findings can be simply carried over to people with Type 1 diabetes. Similarly, the tools used to quantify arterial risk in the general population are known not to work well in people with Type 2 diabetes, and seem even less likely to be valid in Type 1 diabetes.

▷   Evidence statements

Arterial risk factors

The Scottish intercollegiate guidelines[174] identify specific risk factors for arterial disease as cigarette smoking, dyslipidaemia, hypertension, hyperglycaemia, obesity and micro-albuminuria (**IV**).

The guideline[174] reports on non-randomised studies showing that smoking is an independent arterial risk factor in people with diabetes. Additional observational studies reported dyslipidaemia. An increased concentration of LDL cholesterol or total cholesterol has also been identified as an independent risk factor for arterial morbidity and mortality and each 1.0 mmol/l reduction of LDL cholesterol represents a 36% reduction in risk of arterial disease (**IIa**).

Two controlled but not randomised studies reported within the guideline[174] demonstrated the positive relationship between hypertension and risk of arterial death, with a progressive increase in risk with rising systolic pressure. Each 10 mmHg reduction in systolic pressure is associated with a 15% (95% CI: 12–18) reduction in risk of arterial death over 10 years (**IIa**).

The link between glycaemia and arterial morbidity and mortality was also reported in two studies reviewed in the SIGN guidelines.[174] In one study each 1% reduction in HbA$_{1c}$ was associated with a 21% (95% CI: 15–27) reduction in the risk of diabetes-related death and a 14% reduction for myocardial infarction over 10 years (**IIa**).

Evidence for the other risk factors is sparse. In the SIGN guidelines,[174] no studies were identified for linking obesity as an independent risk factor in established diabetes. One observational study reported microalbuminuria as an independent marker associated with doubling in arterial risk, however, there is insufficient evidence to determine whether reducing albumin excretion rate specifically reduces arterial morbidity or mortality (**IIa**).

A meta-analysis[175] aimed at defining risk factors for arterial disease from studies in people with diabetes, showed that, adjusted for age, both total mortality and death from all vascular causes increased significantly with total cholesterol level and systolic blood pressure, and decreased with percentage of women. Duration of diabetes and mean HbA$_{1c}$ were not considered to be associated with mortality. However, this meta-analysis did not contain a critical appraisal of included studies or details of approaches used to ensure study quality before inclusions and should therefore not be used as the basis for clinical recommendations (**IIa**).

Screening tests

One systematic review[176] examined 67 studies, addressing both screening for primary detection of arterial risk factors and treatment of lipid abnormalities in asymptomatic people both with and without diabetes. Reliability and effectiveness of each screening strategy for identifying lipid disorders was investigated, and showed that total cholesterol measurements generally have good reliability, with an analytic variability of less than or equal to 3% and a mean total biologic variability of the order of 6%. A total cholesterol level within 10% of the true value can be determined with two separate measurements, which do not differ significantly between fasting or non-fasting venous blood (**III**).

Evidence within this systematic review[176] for HDL cholesterol showed a higher analytical (6%) and biological (7.5%) variation than total cholesterol, however, two or three values were required to estimate true HDL cholesterol levels to within 10 to 15%. Variations were also found between non-fasting and fasting blood samples as HDL cholesterol is 5%–10% lower in the non-fasting state, suggesting that non-fasting measurement may slightly overestimate coronary heart disease risk, but not enough to make accuracy of screening unacceptable (**III**).

Additional studies within this systematic review[176] considered triglyceride screening. Values measured varied by 20%–30% between fasting and non-fasting states. LDL cholesterol is calculated from total and HDL cholesterol and triglycerides measurements and application of the Friedewald equation. However, this equation has been found to be inaccurate at triglyceride levels greater than or equal to 4.5 mmol/l when special techniques must be employed (eg ultracentrifugation) (**III**).

Also considered in this systematic review[176] was the comparable accuracy of total and HDL cholesterol from capillary blood samples. These were found to be less reliable without proper attention to calibration and proper testing techniques. One study found that a Framingham-based coronary risk model was the best predictor of IHD mortality. Guidelines reported in the review concluded that the LDL:HDL cholesterol and the total:HDL cholesterol ratios performed equally well in determining arterial outcomes, and the least accurate screening test was that of measuring total cholesterol alone (**III**).

Other studies included in this review[176] assessing characteristics of the screening tests showed that non-fasting total cholesterol alone is the easiest to perform for the patient and provider. Total:HDL cholesterol ratio is easy for patients to obtain and for providers to interpret and performs equally accurately as the LDL:HDL cholesterol ratio strategy. However, one study in the review demonstrated that risk-based algorithms which directly incorporate age, other risk factors and measures of total and HDL cholesterol are the most accurate approach to screening. These processes are difficult to access and so supplemental tables, such as the Sheffield table, can improve the feasibility of a risk-based strategy (**III**).

There was no evidence from this systematic review[176] to inform the question of appropriate frequency of screening. National guidelines recommend a five-year interval for people with previous normal results and more frequent screening in those with borderline values (**IV**).

Prediction of arterial risk

Six studies all published by the same group addressed the relative specificity and sensitivity of the different methods for predicting arterial risk (Sheffield, Modified Sheffield, Joint British Guidelines, Canadian, Framingham categorical, New Zealand, and Joint European guidelines, but not including the UKPDS risk engine).

One study[177] comparing the Sheffield tables to the computer-calculated Framingham equation revealed a low sensitivity and specificity for the Sheffield tables (35% (95% CI 28 to 42) and 98% (95% CI 97 to 99) respectively). The old tables only included patients with systolic blood pressure <160 mmHg, and cholesterol greater than 5.5 mmol/l. Adopting these exclusion criteria led to a substantial reduction in the number of patients eligible for screening without improving detection of risk assessment (**DS**).

Another evaluation[178] studied all seven guidelines against the calculated Framingham equation in 906 people with diabetes, showing Modified Sheffield tables have higher sensitivity (95% *vs* 37%) with a slight reduction in specificity (90% *vs* 97%) compared with the original tables, with a slightly better positive predictive value than the original version (80% *vs* 71%). The Joint British tables have good specificity (99%), but low sensitivity (77%) but the tables perform well at the lower CHD risk of greater than or equal to 15% over 10 years (specificity 92%, sensitivity 96%). Canadian tables perform poorly at the ≥30% risk, and only slightly better at the greater than or equal to 15% level of risk (specificity 100%, sensitivity 5%, and 85% and 98%, respectively). The Framingham categorical tables have a lower specificity (83%) for the identification of high-risk individuals (although risk is greater than or equal to 27% not greater than or equal to 30%) and this deteriorates for identification of those at ≥15% risk (specificity 77%). New Zealand tables had a sensitivity of 69% and specificity of 88% at a greater than or equal to 20% level of risk, at the ≥10% level of risk, specificity deteriorates to 58%. The Joint European tables have a sensitivity of 89% for risk levels greater than or equal to 20% but specificity of only 71%. This means that one in four patients would be incorrectly identified as having a risk above the 20% threshold (**DS**).

A further study from the same investigators[179] assessed the PROCAM program against that of the Framingham equation. Only 56% of the study population were eligible for evaluation with PROCAM. This evaluation also systematically underestimates risk in comparison with the Framingham equation at low levels of absolute risk but overestimates at higher risk levels (**DS**).

The sensitivity and specificity of various risk prediction tables and charts was also investigated in one comparative study.[180] Compared to the Framingham equation the Sheffield tables had a low sensitivity (40% eligible for cholesterol lowering treatment would be identified), but with high specificity and thus low false positive rates. The New Zealand tables had similar sensitivities and specificities to the Sheffield tables, but a 10% level of risk prediction of five-year arterial disease risk threshold specificity is significantly lower than the Sheffield tables. The European tables have better sensitivity than Sheffield and New Zealand tables but specificity is significantly worse than other risk assessment levels leading to an equally low sensitivity. The joint British Societies table has significantly better specificities at greater than or equal to 15% and greater than or equal to 30% 10-year CHD risk than the modified Sheffield tables. Sensitivity is generally low, but high at the 15% 10-year CHD/10% five-year CVD risk level. Canadian tables are not reliable at greater than or equal to 30% risk but are comparable with the modified Sheffield tables at 154% risk threshold. The Framingham equation had the best performance with sensitivity and specificity comparable to that of the modified Sheffield and joint British Society methods, respectively (**DS**).

▷ Consideration

The group recognised the very considerable difficulties in reaching conclusions from the evidence in this area. Very little direct information pertaining to people with Type 1 diabetes can be ascertained, whilst the importance of the issue is emphasised by the very high early arterial disease (CVD) risk run by people with Type 1 diabetes. Nevertheless certain sub-groups are known to be at particularly high risk (people with raised albumin excretion rate (micro-albuminuria)), while others combine Type 1 diabetes with combinations of classic risk factors typical of the metabolic syndrome and known to be predictors of high arterial risk in people with Type 2 diabetes and indeed non-diabetic populations. A further group of people will combine Type 1 diabetes with a single arterial risk factor or risk marker, while yet others will have Type 1 diabetes but appear low risk otherwise.

Accordingly the important factors for surveillance are urinary albumin excretion (most important), other classical risk factors including full lipid profile, and risk markers such as age, family history and some ethnic groups. In accordance with the principle of unified organisation of care, monitoring of these factors annually is to be recommended, but it was recognised that in low risk individuals technology might become capable of programming longer review intervals for serum lipids.

The group recognised that different ways of using information from a full lipid profile (calculated LDL and HDL separately, calculation of total: HDL cholesterol ratio, calculation of non-HDL cholesterol) are in use. While the group preferred the first of these as not mixing lipid abnormalities of different pathogenesis, and being a better route to using the treatments for different lipid disorders rationally, it was recognised that there was not good evidence to suggest supporting one approach over the others.

The group could find no confidence in any risk table, engine or equation when applied to people with Type 1 diabetes.

RECOMMENDATIONS

R84   Arterial risk factors should be assessed annually, and the assessment should include: C
- albumin excretion rate
- smoking
- blood glucose control
- blood pressure
- full lipid profile (including HDL and LDL cholesterol and triglycerides)
- age
- family history of arterial disease (CVD)
- abdominal adiposity.

R85   Arterial risk tables, equations or engines for calculation of arterial risk should not be   DS
used because they underestimate risk in adults with Type 1 diabetes.

R86   Adults with raised albumin excretion rate (microalbuminuria), or two or more features   **D**
of the metabolic syndrome (see Table 4), should be managed as the highest risk
category (as though they had Type 2 diabetes or declared arterial disease).

Table 4 Features of the metabolic syndrome suggesting high arterial risk in people with Type 1 diabetes		
Feature	Women	Men
Blood pressure average (mmHg)	>135/80	>135/80
Waist circumference (m) *(use 0.10m lower figures for people of South Asian extraction)*	>0.90	>1.00
Serum HDL cholesterol (mmol/l)	<1.2	<1.0
Serum triglycerides (mmol/l)	>1.8	>1.8

Raised albumin exrection rate is not included because in Type 1 diabetes it is a marker of developing nephropathy and nephropathy alone is associated with extreme risk of ischaemic heart disease.
Glucose intolerance cannot be assessed in adults with Type 1 diabetes, but higher insulin doses in adults >20 years (>1.0 U/kg/day) suggest insulin insensitivity.

R87   Adults with Type 1 diabetes who are not in the highest risk category but who have   **D**
other arterial risk factors (increasing age over 35 years, family history of premature heart
disease, of ethnic group with high risk or with more severe abnormalities of blood
lipids or blood pressure) should be managed as a moderately high risk group.

R88   Where there is no evidence of additional arterial risk, the management of lipids and   **D**
blood pressure should follow normal procedures for the non-diabetes population, using
appropriate clinical guidelines.

8.2   Interventions to reduce risk and to manage arterial disease

▷   Rationale

Prevention of arterial risk in people with Type 1 diabetes, through attention to blood glucose
control (insulin therapy, patient education, nutrition, self-monitoring) is considered elsewhere
in this guideline, and blood pressure management in 8.3, below. However, in the general
population (at much lower risk) and in people with Type 2 diabetes other therapies are known
to reduce the risk of arterial events. The current section therefore deals with these approaches
as applied to people with Type 1 diabetes.

▷   Evidence statements

Lipid lowering therapy

The Scottish intercollegiate guidelines[174] identify a role for lipid-lowering drugs in reducing
ischaemic heart disease events but not all cause mortality in people with no known arterial
disease, compared with placebo (**Ia**).

SIGN guidelines on lipids[181] and the prevention of ischaemic heart disease detail studies
targeted at people with Type 2 diabetes. However, secondary prevention trials of lipids reported

in the guideline have shown significant reduction in arterial disease in both Type 1 and Type 2 diabetes. These guidelines recommend the loss of weight, reduction of intake of saturated fat, increased consumption of fruit and vegetables, regular exercise and the introduction of lipid-lowering drug treatment for primary prevention of arterial problems in high-risk people with diabetes. The guidelines also report a study raising concern about underestimating diabetic ischaemic heart disease risk, particularly in people with Type 1 diabetes (**Ia**).

The SIGN guidelines[174] report on a number of therapeutic studies. The CARE study demonstrated a significant reduction in coronary events with pravastatin *vs* placebo, although the magnitude of effect was lower than in the 4S study. The LIPID study also showed a trend to reduction in recurrent coronary events but numbers of people with diabetes in this study were too low to demonstrate statistical significance. The VA-HIT study showed significant secondary prevention of coronary events in men with diabetes aged less than 74 years, taking a fibrate (gemfibrozil) for a mean follow-up of 5.1 years (**Ia**).

Three randomised controlled trials[182–184] reported on the positive effect of pravastatin on arterial outcomes in people with diabetes. One study[182] reported a significant change in total and LDL cholesterol, HDL cholesterol and triglycerides *vs* placebo. After 24 weeks the reduction in total cholesterol from baseline was 22%, LDL cholesterol 26%, and triglycerides decreased by 2%, accompanied by an increase in HDL cholesterol of 14%. Pravastatin was well tolerated throughout the study (**Ib**).

Similar results were seen in the further two trials. One study[183] reported reductions in LDL cholesterol and VLDL cholesterol of 30% and 13% respectively with pravastatin compared with placebo and significant increases in HDL cholesterol at eight and 16 weeks. The final study[184] was in a majority of sulfonylurea treated people with Type 2 diabetes, and pravastatin reduced total and LDL cholesterol by 19% and 27% in the diabetes group. Compared with placebo pravastatin caused a 13% decrease in triglycerides and a 4% increase HDL cholesterol in people with diabetes. Results were similar to those in people without diabetes, and were unaffected by adjustment for age and sex (**Ib**).

The SIGN management of arterial disease in diabetes guidelines[174] cite results from the Scandinavian Simvastan study, which contained 204 people with diabetes (of a study population of 4,444), and demonstrated that cholesterol-lowering therapy was highly effective compared with placebo in those undergoing revascularisation procedures, especially in those with diabetes (risk reduction 55% *vs* 32% in non-diabetes) (**Ia**).

Two RCTs reported the effect of simvastatin in people with diabetes. Total and LDL cholesterol levels and the ratio between LDL and HDL cholesterol were decreased following treatment in one study[185] of 25 people with diabetes, whereas no difference was seen following placebo, no between group comparison was made. The second study, containing 26 people with Type 1 diabetes[186] also reported a significant reduction in the plasma concentrations of total cholesterol, LDL cholesterol and apolipoprotein B after 12 weeks simvastatin treatment, whereas no changes were observed after placebo treatment (**Ib**).

One study reported the effect of bezafibrate on arterial outcomes in 36 people with Type 1 diabetes.[187] However, there are some potential methodological limitations in this study, which does not make this evidence a reliable basis for a clinical recommendation (**Ib**).

Antiplatelet therapy

The SIGN guidelines[174] report uncertainty about the role of aspirin in primary prevention. Citing the HOT study (a randomised controlled trial) and the further reduction in arterial risk in well-controlled hypertensive patients with diabetes, they note the importance of balancing this reduction against the risk of bleeding (**Ia**).

The North of England guidelines[188] on aspirin for the secondary prophylaxis of vascular disease in primary care reported a pooled risk ratio by combining he meta-analysis of the Antiplatelet Collaborative Group with trials published after 1990 to establish the impact of antiplatelet therapy on subsequent myocardial infarction (MI), stroke and vascular death. This provided strong evidence for a general protective effect of aspirin as antiplatelet therapy in patients at raised vascular risk. Few studies were found containing comparisons of aspirin and alternative antiplatelet agents to enable comparison of their relative effectiveness (**Ia**).

For evidence relating specifically to people with diabetes the North of England guidelines[188] identified eight trials contributing to an overall estimate of risk difference for arterial morbidity of 1.2% with aspirin compared to placebo or other antiplatelet agent. These trials were homogeneous with a pooled incidence rate difference (by random effects model) of a 0.3% reduction in the risk of MI, stroke or vascular death from antiplatelet therapy for one year. This is not a statistically significant difference, and in summary authors state that aspirin given to patients with diabetes appears to have a small and statistically uncertain effect upon the risk of experiencing a subsequent vascular event. They also suggest that the similar relative risk for MI, stroke and vascular death found in diabetes trials and other trials of patients at raised vascular risk, indicates that patients with diabetes alongside other indications of vascular risk are likely to benefit from routine aspirin therapy (**Ia**).

American Diabetes Association guidelines[76] indicate that meta-analysis and large-scale collaborative trials in men and women with diabetes support the view that low-dose aspirin therapy should be prescribed as a secondary prevention strategy if no contraindications exist. The guidelines also point to substantial evidence suggesting that low-dose aspirin therapy should be used as a primary prevention strategy in men and women with diabetes who are at a high risk for arterial events.

The meta-analysis of 145 prospective controlled trials of antiplatelet therapy by the Antiplatelet Trialists Group reported in the ADA guidelines[76] showed a trend toward increased risk reductions with doses of aspirin ≤325 mg/day, but the difference was not statistically significant. An estimated 38±12 vascular events per 1,000 patients with Type 1 diabetes would have been prevented if they were treated with aspirin as a secondary prevention strategy (**Ia**).

The ADA guidelines[76] also reported on the HOT study, which showed a reduction in arterial events following aspirin therapy compared to placebo of 15% and a 36% reduction in myocardial infarction. This study also showed that fatal bleeding including intracerebral bleeding were equal in aspirin and control groups, whereas non-fatal minor bleeding episodes were more frequent in patients receiving aspirin. The US Physicians Health study reported in the same guideline compared aspirin (325 mg/day) with placebo in male physicians (without diabetes), resulting in a 44% risk reduction in MI among the treated group. In a subgroup of people with diabetes there was a reduction in MI from 10% to 4% yielding a relative risk of 0.39 for men with diabetes randomised to aspirin therapy (**Ia**).

The ADA guidelines[76] also addressed the safety of aspirin use and reported several prospective randomised studies in which a trend for an increase in haemorrhagic stroke followed aspirin therapy, although this has not reached statistical significance (**Ia**).

Contraindications reported[76] include allergy, bleeding tendency, anticoagulant therapy, recent gastrointestinal bleeding and clinically active hepatic disease (**Ib**).

Relative risk of MI reported by the ETDRS group[189] in which roughly 48% of men and women with diabetes had a history of arterial disease was lowered significantly in the first five years in those randomised to aspirin therapy (**Ib**).

In the management of people with diabetes and new or established vascular disease, the SIGN guidelines[174] refer to a meta-analysis of platelet inhibitor therapy demonstrating a 31% reduction in non-fatal reinfarction, a 42% reduction in non-fatal stroke and a 13% reduction in arterial mortality (**Ia**).

One meta-analysis[190] of six randomised, double-blind, placebo-controlled trials showed a significant pooled reduction in mortality following treatment with platelet glycoprotein inhibitors. The most marked benefit was seen in patients undergoing percutaneous coronary intervention. A significant reduction in composite death or MI at 30 days was also seen following treatment in people with diabetes. However, potential methodological limitations of the trials included would not permit this analysis to be used as a evidence base to inform recommendations in this area (**Ia**).

Also reported in the SIGN guideline[174] is a sub-study analysis of a large RCT demonstrating that addition of clopidogrel to aspirin over 3–12 months reduces the risk of fatal or non-fatal MI or stroke by 20% in patients with a past history of coronary heart disease presenting with acute coronary syndromes (without electrocardiographic ST elevation). This risk reduction was however associated with an additional risk of bleeding (**Ia**).

The ADA guidelines[76] also report from the CAPRIE study which showed that clopidogrel was slightly more effective than aspirin in reducing the combined risk of stroke, MI or vascular death in people with and without diabetes (effect sizes not stated) (**Ia**).

Management of arterial disease

One randomised controlled study reviewed in the ADA guideline[76] showed that thrombolytic therapy reduced mortality after acute MI in subjects with diabetes by ≤42% with no increase in risk of bleeding or stroke, and should not be withheld due to concern about retinal haemorrhage in patients with retinopathy. This study also demonstrated that the indications and contraindications for thrombolysis in patients with diabetes are the same as those without (**Ia**).

The SIGN guideline[174] reports on the results of the beta-blocker adrenergic pooling project study, which demonstrated that diabetes is not a contraindication to the use of beta-blockers, and that these reduce mortality, sudden cardiac death and re-infarction when given after acute MI. The guideline also cites the 1995 Collaborative Group on ACE inhibitor trials meta-analysis of nearly 100,000 patients which showed that receiving therapy with an ACE inhibitor within 36 hours of acute MI for ≥4 weeks, reduced mortality post MI. The majority of benefits occurred within the first few days when mortality was highest, benefiting patients at a higher risk to a greater absolute extent (**Ia**).

Three large trials (AIRE, SAVE and TRACE studies)[174] also reviewed within the SIGN guideline have shown consistent reductions in mortality when ACE inhibitor therapy is given to people after acute MI with clinical evidence of heart failure or a reduced ejection fraction. A fourth study (SOLVD) demonstrated an absolute risk reduction for mortality of 4.5% in patients with diabetes and chronic heart failure given an ACE inhibitor compared to placebo over a mean follow-up of 4.5 years (**Ia**).

A predefined subgroup analysis of 3,577 people over 55 with diabetes (the majority of whom had Type 2 diabetes) in the large multinational HOPE randomised controlled trial[191] showed the effect of ramipril on arterial outcomes in people with diabetes. The rate of combined primary outcome of MI, stroke or arterial death was significantly lower in the ramipril groups than in those receiving placebo. Total mortality was reduced by 24%. Adjustment for changes in systolic and diastolic blood pressures did not change the magnitude of the effect (**Ib**).

Other results from the HOPE study[192] in which patients aged over 55 years, with and without diabetes, who were randomised to receive 400 IU vitamin E for an average follow-up of 4.5 years, showed no effect of antioxidant over placebo. Primary outcomes of MI, stroke or arterial death, or secondary outcomes of hospitalisations for angina or heart failure, were similar following treatment with vitamin E and placebo. No differences were observed in the frequency of outcomes in people with diabetes in the two treatment groups (**Ib**).

Management of acute stroke

SIGN guidelines[174] state that clinical presentation of stroke in people with diabetes is similar to that in people without diabetes. There is little evidence specific to people with diabetes let alone specific to Type 1 diabetes, suggesting that the management of stroke should be similar to that in people without diabetes (**IV**).

▷ Health economic evidence

Whilst economic analyses have been conducted on trials of lipid-lowering agents, no evaluation has specifically considered Type 1 diabetes. Three papers were identified within the health economic literature dealing with mixed diabetic populations.[350–52] An economic analysis[350] of simvastatin using the 4S trial data suggests that it would provide cost-effective mortality reduction in the UK amongst a similar population. A second cost-effectiveness paper[351] also suggests that the simvastatin may be cost-effective in the UK for those aged 40 to 70 years with elevated cholesterol even if they have not been diagnosed with arterial disease. A third paper based outside the UK suggests that the benefits of simvastatin to diabetics with elevated lipid levels and arterial disease outweigh the benefit to those with elevated lipid levels and no prior arterial disease.[352]

As the GDG has no confidence in any existing risk table, engine or equation when applied to those with Type 1 diabetes, the degree to which models that make use of such equations can be relied upon is extremely limited.

▷ Consideration

The data on arterial risk management in people with Type 1 diabetes are few, though it is noted that studies in people with and without Type 2 diabetes point to clinically effective interventions for those groups. In the absence of quantitative risk assessment and noting the economic evidence placed before the group it seemed clear that interventions in people with Type 1 diabetes must be recommended considering their semi-quantitative arterial disease risk: high, moderate or no risk.

Given the high arterial risk of many people with Type 1 diabetes, smoking was considered to be particularly disadvantageous.

RECOMMENDATIONS

These recommendations assume that arterial risk has been assessed according to the recommendations in section 8.1. Blood glucose control, blood pressure control and education programmes are considered elsewhere in this guideline (see 7, 8.3, 6.1 respectively).

R89	Adults with Type 1 diabetes who smoke should be given advice on smoking cessation and use of smoking cessation services, including NICE guidance-recommended therapies. The messages should be reinforced in continuing smokers yearly if pre-contemplative of stopping, and at all clinical contacts if there is a prospect of their stopping.	D
R90	Young adult non-smokers should be advised never to start smoking.	D
R91	Aspirin therapy (75 mg daily) should be recommended in adults in the highest and moderately-high risk categories.	B
R92	A standard dose of a statin should be recommended for adults in the highest risk and moderately-high risk groups. Therapy should not be stopped if alanine aminotransferase (ALT) is raised to less than three times the upper limit of reference range.	B
R93	If several statins are not tolerated, fibrates and other lipid-lowering drugs should be considered as indicated according to assessed arterial risk status.	D
R94	Fibrates should be recommended for adults with hypertriglyceridaemia according to local lipid-lowering guidelines, and arterial disease risk status.	D
R95	Responses to therapy should be monitored by assessment of lipid profile. If the response is unsatisfactory, the following causes should be considered: non-concordance, inappropriate drug choice and the need for combination therapy.	D
R96	Adults who have had myocardial infarction or stroke should be managed intensively, according to relevant non-diabetes guidelines. In the presence of angina or other ischaemic heart disease, β-adrenergic blockers should be considered (for use of insulin in these circumstances, see R165.)	D

8.3 Blood pressure

▷ Rationale

Blood pressure is an accepted arterial risk factor. Some drugs used in blood pressure management have been suggested as having metabolic effects or interacting with insulin therapy. Accordingly blood pressure management in people with Type 1 diabetes might be different from people who do not have diabetes. However, those with developing diabetic kidney disease may have different needs again, and are considered separately in chapter 10.

▷ Evidence statements

Drug therapy

A significant amount of research has been conducted into the treatment of hypertension in recent years. Primary endpoints for this research are the reduction of arterial and microvascular complications by the reduction of blood pressure to within target levels.

Three sets of national clinical guidelines have been published in the last two years – Canadian,[193] American,[76] and Scottish[194] – presenting rigorous systematic reviews of evidence in this area to date.

The UKPDS[195] randomised controlled trial (in people with Type 2 diabetes) showed that lowering blood pressure in people with diabetes reduces the risk of macrovascular and microvascular disease (**Ib**).

British Hypertension Society guidelines[196] recommend a threshold for initiating antihypertensive treatment in people with diabetes at ≥140/90 mmHg. Target blood pressure for this group of people is advised at <140/80 mmHg unless nephropathy or proteinuria (>1 g/24h) is present when this target is lowered to <130/80 mmHg and <127/75 mmHg, respectively. The guidelines also recommend that blood pressure reduction and ACE inhibitors can be employed to reduce the rate of decline in renal function in people with hypertension and diabetic nephropathy (**IV**).

British Hypertension Society guidelines[196] suggest that treatment should essentially be the same in people with Type 1 and Type 2 diabetes. Several studies are cited which provide evidence for the safety and efficacy of ACE inhibitors, dihydropyridine calcium channel blockers, low dose thiazide diuretics and β-adrenergic blockers in the treatment of hypertension in people with diabetes. The guidelines recommend that the choice among these drug classes should be determined using the criteria set out for people without diabetes (**IV**).

The large multicentre randomised ALLHAT trial[197] showed no superiority of a calcium channel blocker (amlodipine) or an ACE inhibitor (lisinopril) over a thiazide diuretic (chlorthalidone) in preventing major coronary events or in increasing survival in older people both with and without Type 2 diabetes. This RCT of long duration[197] found that lisinopril therapy had a 15% higher risk for stroke and a 10% higher risk of combined CVD compared to chlorthalidone in a mixed population with 36% of people with diabetes. The six-year absolute risk difference for combined CVD was 2.4%, which included a 19% higher risk of heart failure and 10% higher risk of hospitalised/fatal heart failure (not statistically significant), also a 11% higher risk for treated angina and 10% higher risk of coronary revascularisation were statistically significant outcomes. Patients assigned to amlodipine had a 38% higher risk of heart failure, a six-year absolute risk difference of 2.5% and a 35% higher risk of fatal heart failure compared to those on chlorthalidone. Further long-term outcomes reported in this study showed that diuretic was superior to the calcium channel blocker in preventing major coronary events or increasing survival, although their effect on overall CVD prevention was comparable. Diuretic treatment was superior to ACE inhibitor lowering of blood pressure and in preventing aggregate arterial events (mainly stroke, heart failure, angina and coronary revascularisation) in both people with and without Type 2 diabetes (**Ib**).

Two meta-analyses of randomised controlled trials cited in the Scottish guidelines,[194] demonstrated that thiazides, beta-blockers, ACE inhibitors and calcium channel blockers are all effective in lowering blood pressure and reducing the risk of arterial events (**Ia**).

A large randomised controlled study of the use of an angiotensin II receptor antagonist compared to a β-adrenergic blocker in people with diabetes (predominantly Type 2 diabetes) found the angiotensin II receptor antagonist significantly reduced the risk of arterial mortality or stroke, and MI over four or more years of follow-up (**Ia**).

Randomised controlled trials reported within the SIGN guidelines[194] state that combination therapy is often required to reach target blood pressure, either with the same class of drug or in combination with another type of drug. The superiority of one combination regimen over another has not been examined or documented in Type 1 diabetes (**Ia**).

Several trials report the benefit of ACE inhibitors in producing highly significant and clinically important reductions in endpoints of MI, stroke and arterial death.

Multiple trials and systematic reviews[76,174,193,198] have consistently demonstrated substantial benefits from ACE inhibitors in people with Type 1 diabetes with hypertension and diabetic nephropathy. In diabetic nephropathy these antihypertensives reduce progression from micro- to macroalbuminuria and to end stage renal disease compared to placebo as reported in a well developed systematic review[193] (**Ia**).

Two sets of SIGN guidelines[174,194] recommend ACE inhibitors as first-line therapy in patients with microalbuminuria due to their additional benefit on renal function, based on a review of RCT-based evidence (**Ia**).

Adverse effects of ACE inhibitors described in clinical trials and found to be problematic in clinical use include a persistent cough (**IV**).

The ADA technical review[76] and one randomised controlled study in the Canadian guidelines[193] suggest that if ACE inhibitors are prescribed, serum creatinine and potassium levels should be measured at baseline and one to two weeks after initiation (**Ia**).

The UKPDS showed apparent equivalence of beta-blockers (atenolol) with ACE inhibitors (captopril) to moderate blood pressure in people with diabetic nephropathy; this study was in people with Type 2 diabetes and had insufficient power to show any change of clinical significance[174] (**Ia**).

Three randomised studies have shown similar reductions in proteinuria in diabetic antihypertensive patients with beta-blockers and ACE inhibitors as reported in a systematic review[76] (**Ia**).

Concern around the blunting of recovery from hypoglycaemia by beta-blockers was not confirmed in a large randomised study on people with Type 2 diabetes, but caution is urged when prescribing to insulin-treated people with a history of severe hypoglycaemia[76] (**Ia**).

There is no robust evidence to recommend the use of alpha-blockers as first-line treatment in antihypertensive therapy. One ongoing multicentre trial is reported in a systematic review as having discontinued the alpha-blocker arm of the study due to increased incidence of arterial events in this treatment group[76] (**Ia**).

A recent meta-analysis suggests that dihydropyridine calcium channel blockers may be equivalent in protecting against stroke, but less effective in reducing MI and coronary events than ACE inhibitors, beta-blockers or diuretics[76] (**Ia**).

One randomised study[199] found no difference between dihydropyridine calcium channel blockers and other antihypertensive drugs with respect to diabetic nephropathy. In addition, the American guidelines[76] urge caution as it is difficult to compare trials studying different calcium channel blockers due to their diverse pharmacological effects (**Ia**).

Evidence for the use of thiazide diuretics is not as robust as for other antihypertensive therapies.[193] Treatment has been associated with hypokalaemia, hyponatraemia, volume depletion, hypercalcaemia and hyperuricaemia. Two retrospective studies reported in the American guidelines[76] suggested increased arterial mortality, and other studies have shown that thiazides may not be as effective in subjects with significantly decreased renal function (**IV**).

Target blood pressure

Two large multicentre trials included in a systematic review[193] showed an improvement in arterial and microvascular outcome in patients randomised to lower target blood pressures compared to those with less intensive blood pressure lowering. Evidence supports a treatment goal of diastolic BP <80 mmHg (**Ia**).

No evidence exists on the appropriate target systolic blood pressure for people with Type 1 diabetes. Consensus recommendations from the Canadian Hypertension Recommendations working group[193] is that systolic blood pressure should be <130mmHg (**IV**).

The SIGN hypertension guidelines[194] note that RCTs use target blood pressures of <130/80 mmHg in major outcome trials or 125/75 mmHg when proteinuria >1g/24h is present (**IV**).

Behavioural therapy

A rigorous systematic review performed in the production of the American Diabetes Association guidelines[76] on the treatment of hypertension in diabetes reported one meta-analysis of RCTs showing that dietary management with moderate sodium restriction has been effective in reducing blood pressure in individuals with essential hypertension. However, this has not been tested in a diabetic population. No evidence exists for significant benefit of magnesium supplementation or calcium supplementation in people with diabetes (**Ia**).

Weight reduction has also been shown in a systematic review of non-randomised controlled trials[76] to reduce blood pressure independently of sodium intake and to improve glucose and lipid levels (**IIa**).

Smoking cessation, moderation of alcohol intake and mild physical activity have been recommended by the Joint National Committee on Prevention, Detection, Evaluation and Treatment of High Blood Pressure to reduce blood pressure[76] (**IV**).

The American Diabetes Association guidelines[76] recommend that patients with a systolic blood pressure of 130–139 or diastolic blood pressure of 80–89 mmHg should be given lifestyle/behavioural therapy as first-line treatment for a maximum of three months, based on evidence from large scale RCTs (**Ia**).

▷   Health economic evidence

The health economic literature on Type 1 diabetes does not assess the cost-effectiveness of ACE inhibitors in lowering blood pressure in isolation. The effect of ACE inhibitors in lowering blood pressure is linked in these studies to its effects in delaying kidney damage, and the GDG felt that no recommendations in regard of blood pressure lowering alone could be drawn from the existing evidence.

▷   Consideration

The finding of raised blood pressure in people with diabetes is felt to be of different significance in the presence of nephropathy, if features of the metabolic syndrome are present, or in the absence of these findings. Other risk factors (age, ethnic group, family history, smoking) will be relevant in the last group, in whom it was felt management should echo that of non-diabetic people of the same age, but regarding the diabetes as a further substantial risk factor. (Formal risk calculation was considered above under arterial disease surveillance, and is not recommended.) The combination of raised blood pressure and nephropathy or features of the metabolic syndrome is however known to be very high risk indeed for premature arterial disease in early middle age. Accordingly intervention levels and targets should be lower and more strictly applied than for the person with 'simple' hypertension. Very many suggestions for intervention levels based on evidence have been put forward by other groups, with (allowing for the gradual evolution of evidence) considerable coherence. The group assessed all the available recommendations in this area and reached a consensus based on small differences between these.

The problems of motivating professionals and people with diabetes to manage blood pressure appropriately, despite the clear arterial and macrovascular protection to be gained, were noted to be multifactorial. Accordingly, recommendations emphasising intervention levels, targeting, informed discussions and patient-held record cards were discussed. The problem of potential and minor side effects inhibiting the achievement of major clinical gains was felt to be worth mentioning. It was noted that lifestyle interventions have a role in blood pressure management (considered in more detail in other parts of this guideline).

RECOMMENDATIONS

R97   Intervention levels for recommending blood pressure management should be   D
135/85 mmHg unless the person with Type 1 diabetes has abnormal albumin excretion rate or two or more features of the metabolic syndrome (see Table 4), in which case it should be 130/80 mmHg. See also R116–18.

R98   To allow informed choice by the person with the condition, the following should be   D
discussed:

- reasons for choice of intervention level
- substantial potential gains from small improvements in blood pressure control
- possible negative consequences of therapy.

See also R116–18 in chapter 10.

R99   A trial of a low-dose thiazide diuretic should be started as first-line therapy for raised   D
blood pressure, unless the person with Type 1 diabetes is already taking a renin-
angiotensin system blocking drug for nephropathy (see Chapter 10). Multiple drug
therapy will often be required.

R100   Adults with Type 1 diabetes should be offered information on the potential for lifestyle   D
changes to improve blood pressure control and associated outcomes, and offered
assistance in achieving their aims in this area.

R101   Concerns over potential side effects should not be allowed to inhibit advising and   D
offering the necessary use of any class of drugs, unless the side effects become
symptomatic or otherwise clinically significant. In particular:

- selective β-adrenergic blockers should not be avoided in adults on insulin
- low-dose thiazides may be combined with beta-blockers
- when calcium channel antagonists are prescribed, only long-acting preparations should be used
- direct questioning should be used to detect the potential side effects of erectile dysfunction, lethargy and orthostatic hypotension with different drug classes.

9 Management of late complications: diabetic eye disease

9.1 Retinopathy surveillance programmes

▷ Rationale

Diabetes eye damage is the single largest cause of blindness before old age. The success of laser therapy in the treatment of sight-threatening retinopathy is an accepted part of ophthalmological care and has not been assessed for this guideline. Appropriate issues which need to be addressed are, however, how people with developing retinopathy can be selected for ophthalmological referral in time for optimal treatment, and whether preventative therapy other than good blood glucose and good blood pressure control can be useful in people with Type 1 diabetes. This section deals with the structure and success of surveillance programmes, while the methods used for detection of early retinopathy, the use of alternative preventative therapies and referral guidelines to ophthalmology are considered below.

▷ Evidence statements

The SIGN guideline[174] suggested from two comparative studies that screening is effective at detecting unrecognised sight-threatening retinopathy. Onset of pre-proliferative retinopathy was identified in one study 3.5 years after diagnosis of Type 1 diabetes in post-puberty patients, and within two months of onset of puberty (IIa).

There are discrepancies in the recommended optimal frequency of testing for diabetic retinopathy. Annual review was considered appropriate by consensus in two guidelines.[174,200] Testing for other diabetic complications takes place annually, and this is considered an appropriate schedule for retinopathy screening (IV).

The NICE guidelines for Type 2 diabetes[201] reached consensus on a more frequent need for screening (three to six months) in patients who experienced worsening of lesions or scattered exudates more than one disc diameter from the fovea or in a person with changes in blood glucose control suggesting higher risk of progression of retinopathy (NICE).

Further research is needed in increasing this screening interval for low-risk patients. Evidence from non-randomised controlled studies considered in a systematic review found that patients with no retinopathy at baseline have a less than 1% chance of developing any retinopathy within two years[174] (IIa).

Evidence from patient focus groups and the grey literature suggests that success of screening depends on continued consistently high levels of uptake. Patients expressed importance in discussing fear of blindness and benefits of attending regular screening. Explanations of techniques and technologies for screening including new technologies under investigation were requested. The need for eye drops and transient effects on vision should also be communicated. Multiple patient reminders did not improve attendance at screening sessions. A range of education methods is needed to encourage non-attendees (IV).

SIGN guidelines[174] cite cohort studies with high risk of potential confounding in their design and expert opinion indicating that patients prefer screening to be performed at a site convenient to them. Low vision clinics and community self-help groups can improve the quality of life and functional ability of patients with visual impairment. Community support, low vision aids and training, and assistance to register as blind/partially sighted should be provided to people with diabetes and visual impairment (**IV**).

▷ Health economic evidence

The health economic searches produced nine papers of potential interest to the guideline that fall into three distinct sets. The first set of five papers[354–8] present US and Swedish simulations of the cost-effectiveness of the screening for and treatment of diabetic retinopathy using a similar model structure. All these papers consider retinopathy screening at a yearly or more frequent interval. Three of the papers[354–6] relate to a government perspective within the US, where the cost of federal benefits for blindness is argued to be greater than the costs of a yearly (or more frequent) screening regimen for those with retinopathy. A fourth paper relates the model to Sweden,[357] where it is argued that retinopathy screening is cost-saving to the government. A final paper,[358] also US based, considers only medical costs (a health insurer standpoint) and finds a cost-effectiveness ratio of $1,996 per QALY (1990 prices) for the yearly screening of those without retinopathy and a six-monthly screening for those with retinopathy.

Two other related papers[359–60] consider national retinopathy screening using an alternative model. In one of these papers, only minimal glycaemic control is assumed (HbA$_{1c}$ at 10%) when evaluating retinopathy, whilst the other gives insufficient details of the model or alternative strategies to allow analysis. Both papers appear to produce findings consistent with the cost-effectiveness of screening for and treatment of diabetic retinopathy.

None of the above papers consider the potential role of digital photography in detecting diabetic retinopathy at low marginal cost.

Two papers[361–2] consider the screening methods used in dispersed or isolated populations. Of these, one relates to a mixed population with a very low proportion of Type 1 diabetes,[362] whilst the other uses highly-specific cost estimates.[361] As no large dispersed or isolated subgroup exists within the UK, the results of these papers are not relevant for the guideline.

▷ Consideration

Members of the group recognised that some people with long-standing stable eye condition (and unchanging metabolic and blood pressure control) did not necessarily justify annual eye surveillance, but that currently the practicalities and knowledge base for identification and selection and recall of such people meant that a universal minimum recommendation of annually was the correct judgement. More frequent assessment of some individuals with changing retinopathy was noted to be cost-effective as they would otherwise have to be referred to ophthalmologists. The group were aware that future developments in the evidence base may allow for longer intervals between assessments for low-risk individuals. The importance of education of people with diabetes as to the purpose of the surveillance was agreed, while the issue of convenience of site was noted to have significant cost consequences.

RECOMMENDATIONS

R102	Eye surveillance for adults newly diagnosed with Type 1 diabetes should be started from diagnosis.	A

R103 Depending on the findings, structured eye surveillance should be followed by: B
- routine review in one year, or
- earlier review, or
- referral to an ophthalmologist.

R104	Structured eye surveillance should be at one-year intervals.	A

R105 The reasons and success of eye surveillance systems should be properly conveyed to   C
adults with Type 1 diabetes, so that attendance is not reduced by ignorance of need or
fear of outcome.

9.2 Screening tests for retinopathy

▷ Rationale

The success of laser therapy in the treatment of sight-threatening retinopathy is an accepted part of ophthalmological care and has not been assessed for this guideline. The appropriate issue to be addressed is, however, how people with developing retinopathy can be selected for ophthalmological referral in time for optimal treatment. This section deals with the methods used for detection of early retinopathy, the structure of surveillance programmes having been covered in the previous section, while other therapy issues are covered in 9.3.

▷ Evidence statements

Ophthalmoscopy

Direct ophthalmoscopy does not usually meet the required standards for retinopathy screening and review.[201] Sensitivity achieved by GP and optometrist screening with ophthalmoscopes is very low[201–202] (**NICE**).

Ultra-wide angle screening laser ophthalmoscope

Little evidence is available in this area. One comparative study conducted on healthy individuals reported in a systematic review is of limited applicability clinically[202] (**Ia**).

Slit lamp biomicroscopy

A diagnostic study quoted in a systematic review found that slit lamp biomicroscopes with dilated indirect ophthalmoscopy used by properly-trained individuals can achieve sensitivities similar to retinal photography, with a lower technical failure rate[202] (**DS**).

A systematic review concluded that slit lamps are always needed for those not amenable to digital photography[202] (**IV**).

Retinal photography

Retinal cameras have the highest level of accuracy of any practical screening method,[203] and provide permanent images for quality control. Retinal photography is more effective than direct ophthalmoscopy and can regularly achieve a sensitivity of 80%[174] (**DS**).

Photography is more accurate at detecting the presence of microaneurysms than ophthalmoscopy and may be of use in milder disease states[203] (**Ib**).

A low percentage of retinal photographs are ungradeable, although this may be improved by digital imaging. Accuracy is not dependent on the type of professional involved, but data from non-randomised controlled studies underlines the need for training in reading the photographs or images[202] (**IIa**).

Limited evidence exists on the number of fields that should be viewed with a retinal camera. One systematic review[202] considering diagnostic studies showed that single-field studies gave marginally better results than those with two or more fields (**DS**).

Digital cameras show similar accuracy to conventional photography but have advantages in image transfer and potential for automated grading.[202] Technical failure rates are lower with digital cameras (**DS**).

Further evaluation of digital imaging techniques is needed to prove the usefulness of this screening method[174] (**IV**).

There are inconsistent results and conclusions from randomised trials regarding the use of mydriasis in retinal photography reported in a systematic review[202] (**Ia**).

The Health Technology Board for Scotland assessment report[202] states that there is no clear evidence that mydriasis or the routine use of more than one image significantly alters the sensitivity or specificity of screening for the detection of sight-threatening retinopathy. The review concludes that there is little difference between the accuracy and failure rates of modern cameras when used with or without mydriasis; however, the analysis of failure after non-mydriatic photography may have favoured no difference to outcome. Comparable screening accuracy is achieved with digital cameras, with or without mydriasis, however direct comparisons suggest that mydriasis may occasionally result in a successful image when non-mydriatic imaging fails (**DS**).

A large diagnostic study of screening services in both hospital and district settings[204] found screening tests by trained retinal screeners to have a high sensitivity and very high specificity to detect sight-threatening diabetic retinopathy as assessed by slit lamp examination (**DS**).

NICE Type 2 diabetes guidelines[201] suggest that mydriatic 45° retinal photography is the most effective test when screening for diabetic retinopathy (**NICE**).

If more than one image per eye is required for screening then mydriasis is essential because of constriction of the pupil caused by the first photographic flash (**IV**).

Tropicamide (0.5%–1%), administered by a trained professional is a safe and appropriate way to perform mydriasis[174] (**NICE**).

The use of pilocarpine to reduce mydriasis is potentially harmful[202] (**IV**).

Blurred vision and sensitivity to light are complications of the instillation of eye drops for mydriasis. Other related side effects such as glaucoma and allergic reactions are rare[205] (**IV**).

Table 5 Mydriasis with tropicamide

Mydriasis with tropicamide:

- reduces the failure rate (inadequately interpretable photographs) in around 5% of eyes of people with diabetes (in particular in the second eye and in the elderly), and thus the need for recall for a further examination when tropicamide will be necessary

- allows follow-up ophthalmoscopy to be optimised reducing false-negative referrals to ophthalmologists

- carries no detectable risk to the eye except in the post-surgical period

- is briefly uncomfortable (stings)

- paralyses accommodation (near vision) and pupil constriction for 30–60 minutes (low dose), but in some people for much longer, giving problems with glare and bright light sufficient to impair vision to unsafe levels for some tasks (for example driving).

No studies reported whether differences found in sensitivities of healthcare professionals undertaking tests were statistically significant. Comparable sensitivity is achieved by GPs and optometrists using a direct ophthalmoscope through dilated pupils. Optometrists using slit lamp biomicroscopy only achieved moderate sensitivity (62% sensitivity at 95% specificity). The greatest sensitivity was found in comparative studies used in a systematic review with trained graders using mydriatic and non-mydriatic photography[202] (DS).

Initial data indicates that high-resolution automated grading systems compared to conventional grading can identify the absence of microaneurysms on digital images with a high sensitivity[202] (Ia).

A systematic review[202] included a descriptive study evaluating a system for referring photographs to the next level of expertise. Referral when the grader identified any potential sign of retinopathy, with the more experienced professionals involved in the second and third levels, helped maintain effective analysis of images (IV).

Diabetes UK consensus is that an effective screening system should achieve a technical failure rate of less than 5%[206] (IV).

A systematic review[202] reported inconsistent findings from controlled studies of the impact of disease condition and progression of disease on test failure rates (IIa).

Lower technical failure rates are achievable with digital photography compared to conventional slide photography. Failure rates for ophthalmoscopy do not differ greatly from photography in controlled studies reported within a systematic review[202] (IIa).

There is a lack of discrete evidence about the role and usefulness of visual acuity testing. The NICE Type 2 diabetes guideline retinopathy working-group[201] supported the consensus guidelines from the Royal College of Ophthalmologists on the usefulness of visual acuity testing as part of the overall eye care approach (NICE).

Diagnosis of macular oedema rests on the use of stereoscopic, slit lamp, indirect ophthalmoscopy in expert hands. Due to the difficulty of differentiating non-significant and clinically significant macular oedema, the use of visual acuity testing is recommended for screening in routine practice. Reduced visual acuity is an indication for specialist referral[201] (NICE).

▷ Consideration

The group felt that earlier judgements (for example NICE Inherited Type 2 diabetes guideline) that digital photography best met the needs of appropriate sensitivity/selectivity, feasibility and opportunities for quality assurance were clearly endorsed by the evidence review and personal experience of Group members. Mydriasis was noted to be of particular importance in particular groups of people in whom some form of ophthalmoscopy was commonly required to complete a quality examination after photography, and appears safe if inconvenient to some people. It was strongly endorsed. Patient preference studies have suggested that mydriasis may reduce attendance for retinopathy screening because of its temporary effect on vision, but there is no recorded clinical evidence to suggest this. Visual acuity testing, while ill-evidenced, was noted to be fast and non-invasive (though requiring trained staff to test), and provided a useful function in helping detect unsuspected macular oedema, a critical but treatable condition.

RECOMMENDATIONS

R106   Digital retinal photography should be implemented for eye surveillance programmes   **B**
        for adults with Type 1 diabetes.

R107   Mydriasis with tropicamide should be used when photographing the retina,   **B**
        after prior agreement with the person with Type 1 diabetes following discussion of   **D**
        the advantages and disadvantages, including appropriate precautions for driving.

R108   Visual acuity testing should be a routine part of eye surveillance programmes.   **D**

9.3   Referral

▷ Rationale

The issues of surveillance programmes, screening technologies and non-blood glucose/non-blood pressure therapies for prevention are considered in the immediately prior and following sections of this guideline. This section considers the issue of how quickly a person with diabetes should be seen by an ophthalmologist once potentially sight-threatening retinopathy is detected.

▷ Evidence statements

The SIGN guidelines[174] showed from controlled trials that poor outcomes and severe visual loss are associated with a delay in treatment of over two years from diagnosis of sight-threatening diabetic retinopathy. This figure was one year for vitrectomy (**IIa**).

▷ Consideration

The group felt it inappropriate to derive and recommend new referral guidelines without detailed review of the ophthalmological literature, particularly as such guidelines were already published by the Royal College of Ophthalmologists and the National Screening Committee diabetic retinopathy screening group (**www.nscretinopathy.org.uk**). In the area of assessment of macular oedema it was noted that retinal screening recommendations using digital photography (see section 9.2, 'Screening tests for retinopathy') could not inform the referral process suggested by the RCO guideline; thus use of unexplained change in visual acuity was substituted, reflecting current practice.

RECOMMENDATIONS

R109   Emergency review by an ophthalmologist should occur for: D
- sudden loss of vision
- rubeosis iridis
- pre-retinal or vitreous haemorrhage
- retinal detachment.

R110   Rapid review by an ophthalmologist should occur for new vessel formation.   D

R111   Referral to an ophthalmologist should occur for: D
- referable maculopathy:
    - exudate or retinal thickening within one disc diameter of the centre of the fovea
    - circinate or group of exudates within the macula (the macula is defined here as a circle centred on the fovea, of a diameter the distance between the temporal border of the optic disc and the fovea)
    - any microaneurysm or haemorrhage within one disc diameter of the centre of the fovea, only if associated with a best visual acuity of 6/12 or worse
- referable pre-proliferative retinopathy (if cotton wool spots are present, look carefully for the following features, but cotton wool spots themselves do not define pre-proliferative retinopathy):
    - any venous beading
    - any venous loop or reduplication
    - any intraretinal microvascular abnormalities (IRMA)
    - multiple deep, round or blot haemorrhages.
- any unexplained drop in visual acuity.

9.4   Non-surgical treatment of diabetic retinopathy

▷   Rationale

The means and systems of detection of diabetic retinopathy in sufficient time to allow successful laser therapy are considered in the previous three sections. However, laser therapy is a destructive salvage therapy, and prevention by good blood glucose and good blood pressure control are not as yet absolutely successful. Accordingly it is important to consider whether other approaches can delay the development of retinopathy in people with Type 1 diabetes.

▷   Evidence statements

There is a lack of robust evidence for non-surgical, non-laser treatment of diabetic retinopathy. In general, trials in this area have limitations in their methodology.

The SIGN guideline[174] addressed the absence of good evidence for use of ACE inhibitors in diabetic eye disease. One multicentre RCT examined therein is methodologically limited. Trials with ACE inhibitor therapy are ongoing but at present there is inconclusive evidence in this area (**Ia**).

There is limited evidence from trials with the antiplatelet agents ticlopidine[207–208] and dipyridamole[209] that measures for deterioration of retinopathy were significantly lower in patients treated with antiplatelet agents compared to placebo, although potential methodological limitations would prevent this evidence forming the basis of a clinical recommendation. Ticlopidine has a high incidence of side effects (**Ib**).

One three-year study[210] showed a sevenfold reduction in the number of definite annual microaneurysms compared to placebo in insulin-treated patients, and an inverse relationship between progression of microaneurysms and hypo-aggregability level in patients treated with ticlopidine. The trial in this treatment area is of moderate size (**Ib**).

A recent randomised controlled trial[211] showed high dose vitamin E significantly reduced mean circulation time and increased retinal blood flow in diabetic patients. No differences were seen in retinopathy level between the placebo and vitamin E groups (**Ib**).

▷ Consideration

Issues of blood glucose control, blood pressure control or smoking are covered in chapters 7 and 8. Outside these indications the evidence was not felt to be strong enough to justify any recommendation. As this is in line with current practice, no negative recommendations were felt to be needed.

10 Management of late complications: diabetic kidney disease

10.1 Kidney damage

▷ Rationale

Kidney damage in Type 1 diabetes is the largest cause of renal failure in the working age group. Primary prevention by good blood glucose and good blood pressure control is considered elsewhere in this guideline while this section deals with the early detection and management of developing diabetic nephropathy.

▷ Evidence statements

Predictors of nephropathy

One seven-year longitudinal study[212] showed the ability to predict progression to diabetic nephropathy by the presence of microalbuminuria may not be as reliable as previous studies have assumed. Approximately 19% to 24% of patients with microalbuminuria develop diabetic nephropathy. Systolic blood pressure, glycated haemoglobin and triglycerides were significantly higher in people with Type 1 diabetes who progressed to diabetic nephropathy, than for those who did not (**III**).

Five year follow-up[213] of microalbuminuric patients with Type 1 diabetes showed 19% progressed to diabetic nephropathy and 33% regressed to normoalbuminuria. Progressors had significantly higher HbA_{1c} and mean blood pressure and incidence of proliferative retinopathy compared to non-progressors (**III**).

Another seven-year prospective study[214] in 148 normotensive people with diabetes showed that baseline albumin excretion rate (AER) is the predominant predictor for the development of microalbuminuria in Type 1 diabetes. Raised mean arterial blood pressure and HbA_{1c} also were significantly related to progression to microalbuminuria (**III**).

A cohort study of two years follow-up[215] showed in sex-specific analysis that HbA_{1c}, age and baseline AER were particularly important predictors of progression to nephropathy in men, whereas duration of diabetes and triglycerides were particularly important in women. Low-density lipoprotein (LDL) cholesterol was particularly important in people with shorter duration of diabetes and triglycerides in those with a longer diabetes duration (**IIa**).

A case-controlled study with 10-year follow-up[216] showed that baseline glomerular filtration rate (GFR), although not a predictor of end-point AER or microalbuminuria, was a significant predictor of end-of-study blood pressure level. Levels of AER and blood pressure were the main risk factors for renal outcome. A further five-year prospective study[217] showed that in patients with microalbuminuria decline in GFR was independently correlated to onset of diabetic nephropathy and baseline systolic blood pressure (**IIa**).

Screening and diagnosis

The SIGN diabetes guidelines[174] include one comparative study showing that measurements of albumin loss and serum creatinine are the best screening tests for diabetic nephropathy (**III**).

Urine albumin concentration compared to urine albumin:creatinine ratio in a screening accuracy test[218] showed specificity and sensitivity for microalbuminuria of 77% and 82% and 77% and 92% and for macroalbuminuria levels of 84% and 90%, and 88% and 90%. No statistically significant difference was seen when comparing the performance of these two measures in detecting nephropathy (**DS**).

Both albumin concentration and albumin:creatinine ratio measured on a first-pass morning urine sample and compared against timed collection of urinary albumin excretion rate, showed high sensitivity and specificity for normal and elevated albuminuria.[219] Combining the two tests together in the same urine sample revealed the highest sensitivity (98%) and specificity (100%) (**DS**).

A comparative study reported in the SIGN guidelines[174] reports that first-pass morning urine samples best reflect a timed collection and provide adequate assessment of urinary albumin loss (**III**).

One test accuracy study comparing 24-hour urine collection with spot-urine samples[220] showed both samples were accurate for the screening and diagnosis of diabetic nephropathy. Urinary protein better correlates with the reference standard (urinary AER) in macro-albuminuric (0.95) and microalbuminuric (0.80) samples, than in normoalbuminuric samples (0.61) (**DS**).

A 10-year follow up study[221] showed the predication of microalbuminuria is most effective in a four-hour morning urine collection with a greater specificity than 24-hour collection (positive predictive value 91% *vs* 79%), and is similar to the overnight collection, but with a greater sensitivity (**DS**).

One screening test study[222] showed significant intraindividual variation of urinary albumin excretion between samples taken in triplicate for seven days. Mean coefficient of variation was 49%. Urinary albumin excretion >1.0 mg/mmol on the first specimen had a sensitivity of 97% and specificity of 82% for detection of those with a three sample mean >2.5 mg/mmol (**DS**).

A microalbumin analyser was shown in one screening test accuracy study[223] to have sensitivity, specificity, negative predictive and positive predictive values of 92%, 100%, 93% and 100% respectively, suggesting a high reproducibility and reliability for microalbuminuria detection. Another accuracy study[224] showed a different device to have sensitivity, specificity and negative and positive predictive value of 100%, 97%, 100% and 96% respectively (**DS**).

A semi-quantitative diagnostic test[225] reported sensitivity of 86% and specificity of 67% to estimate albumin excretion rate as a screening tool for microalbuminuria. This was considerably lower than the reference standard of albumin concentration (sensitivity 75% and specificity 94%) using the Micral test, which itself is not an effective screening tool for microalbuminuria. A further three studies[226–228] of similar design, predominantly comparing Micral test with urinary albumin excretion rates returned varying results in terms of accuracy. However all suggested a lower sensitivity of Micral test for the detection of albuminuria (**DS**).

One correlation study[229] reporting on self-testing with the Micral test found that 80% of patients classified themselves correctly. Using at least two positive test results increased the specificity and sensitivity to 81% and 92% with a positive predictive value 71% leading to 90% of all patients classifying themselves correctly (III).

One correlation study[230] showed that the dipstick testing method was insensitive or not adequately specific to detect abnormal overnight albumin excretion rate. This study had potential internal validity limitations and should not be used as the basis for a positive clinical recommendation (III).

One diagnostic study[231] of a Clinitek microalbumin test method performed in 302 people with diabetes demonstrated sensitivity and specificity of 79% and 81% and negative and positive predictive values of 46% and 95% for determining microalbuminuria (DS).

Management of nephropathy

The SIGN guideline[174] reports results from the DCCT showing that a reduction in mean HbA_{1c} from 9.0% to 7.3% was associated with a 39% and 54% reduction in the occurrence of microalbuminuria and proteinuria respectively over 6.5 years. However, no clear benefit was seen in the treatment of established microalbuminuria in people with Type 1 diabetes (Ia).

Three prospective studies within the SIGN guideline[174] reported reductions in AER with ACE inhibitors in people with both microalbuminuria and proteinuria. In the former group blood pressure of 112/73 and 122/79 mmHg was associated with a 30% and 18% reduction in AER at 30 and 24 months (Ia).

SIGN guidelines[174] report results from an RCT that ACE inhibitors are more effective than other agents in reducing urinary albumin loss. Three years therapy was associated with a 50% reduction in a combined end-point of death, dialysis or transplantation, this effect was independent of blood pressure (Ia).

A Cochrane systematic review[232] demonstrated the effect of ACE inhibitors on normotensive people with microalbuminuria or overt albuminuria, showing a reduction in albumin excretion rate in patients receiving ACE inhibition compared to placebo. Antihypertensive therapy also reduced blood pressure in treated patients, compared to placebo-treated controls, with no significant effect on GFR or HbA_{1c}. All three ACE inhibitors included in this study had comparable effects (Ia).

A meta-analysis of individual patient data[233] demonstrated a marked benefit in terms of AER being 54% lower in patients receiving ACE inhibitor treatment, compared to those on placebo. Only a small fraction of this effect was due to a decrease in systolic blood pressure. There was a clear gradation in beneficial effect depending on baseline AER. The two-year difference for patients with baseline AER~200 µg/min was 75% compared with 18% in patients with AER ~20 µg/min at baseline (Ia).

A medium-sized randomised controlled trial[234] of 89 normotensive patients failed to show any significant effect of ACE inhibitor treatment on mean arterial BP or creatinine clearance among people with Type 1 diabetes without microalbuminuria followed up for five years (Ib).

Three RCTs compared the effect of ACE inhibitors and calcium channel blockers[235-7] in people with Type 1 diabetes, over follow-up periods of one to four years. One study showed reductions in blood pressure with either agent compared to placebo, but no effect on AER or GFR.[235] The other two studies showed a significantly greater decline in albuminuria in patients treated with the ACE inhibitor, but no other differences between the two treatments.[236–7] Some side effects of calcium channel blockers were seen in all of these studies (**Ib**).

No methodologically robust evidence exists on the use of angiotensin 2 receptor antagonists in the management for nephropathy in people with Type 1 diabetes specifically.

NICE guidelines on Type 2 diabetes[201] report an equally beneficial effect of angiotensin 2 receptor antagonists and ACE inhibitors on renal function in normotensive and hypertensive patients. However, the guidelines comment that the evidence base for angiotensin 2 receptor antagonists is still emerging and caution is urged when making specific recommendations for their use as first-line therapy (**NICE**).

SIGN guidelines[174] recommend angiotensin 2 receptor antagonists should be considered for people with Type 2 diabetes with microalbuminuria or proteinuria (**Ia**).

Two meta-analyses are reported in the SIGN guidelines.[174] These found a reduction of dietary protein to 0.6 to 0.8 g/kg/day was associated with a reduction in the rate of GFR loss in people with proteinuria and impaired renal function, and sensitivity analysis suggested this effect was greater in people with diabetes (**Ia**).

One Cochrane systematic review[238] showed a slight slowing of the decline in GFR following low protein diet for six to 24 months follow-up (mean change in GFR -1.0 and -0.3 (ml/min) for control and treatment groups respectively). All studies included in this review are small and an exact level of protein restriction has yet to be established (**Ia**).

One systematic review[239] that included randomised and non-randomised trials reported eight studies of which some showed significant delay in progression of nephropathy following protein-restricted diets, compared to conventional care. However, some of these studies were methodologically limited by not having sufficient follow-up time to detect particular outcomes (**Ia**).

Two additional RCTs[240–1] were identified in this area. In one study dialysis, transplantation and death occurred in 27% and 10% of patients receiving a usual protein *vs* a low protein diet respectively. Mean blood pressure during follow-up was higher in the usual protein diet group. GFR was comparable between the two groups. The second study found no significant difference in renal function following low protein diet but a significant decrease in body weight and obesity index were seen at the end of 12 months follow-up (**Ib**).

One RCT[242] found no effect of fish oil supplementation on the progression of renal function and albuminuria in normotensive patients with diabetic nephropathy (**Ib**).

Referral

There are no studies directly examining the appropriate timing of referral of people with Type 1 diabetes and diabetic nephropathy to a renal specialist.

Strong explicit consensus in the NICE guidelines[243] for Type 2 diabetes was for specialist referral when serum creatinine is greater than 150 μmol/l (**NICE**).

SIGN guidelines[174] state that although no evidence exists on a time to referral, most renal physicians would prefer patients to be referred earlier rather than later (**IV**).

▷ Health economic evidence

The health economic literature relating to the method of surveillance for emerging kidney damage produced four papers.[363–6] Three of these papers concentrated on the costs of testing, and largely ignored later outcomes. The fourth of these papers[366] presents a cost-utility analysis of laboratory testing *vs* double dipstick testing plus laboratory assays where either result is positive. However, this paper employs a non-standard QALY measure and this limits the robustness of the conclusions.

Five studies[367–71] consider ACE inhibitor use for those found to have proteinuria following screening. One paper[370] was excluded as it was predicated on a significantly different healthcare system than that of the UK. The remaining four papers argued that ACE inhibitor treatment will be cost-saving in those found to exhibit proteinuria.

The cost-effectiveness of ACE inhibitor treatment of those with microalbuminuria[372–5] is also analysed in four papers based outside of the UK, of which two consider benefits from arterial disease in addition to the benefits of delaying or preventing nephropathy.[374–5] Two papers[372,374] suggest ACE inhibitor treatment will be cost-effective on both base case and sensitivity analysis. One cost-utility study[373] (interpretation of which is limited by possible typographic errors in the calculations) considers nephropathy benefits only and suggests ACE inhibitor treatment is cost-effective on their base case analysis but not in sensitivity testing. A final paper considers both nephropathy and arterial benefits and finds a high cost per life year saved.[375]

▷ Consideration

The issue of blood glucose control and its role in the development of microvascular complications is considered elsewhere in this guideline.

While there was no formal evidence on frequency of testing in the individual without previous evidence of nephropathy, organisational issues and the slow time course of progression of nephropathy suggested yearly surveillance in concert with eye and foot surveillance. For perceived reasons of convenience and adherence, spot urine specimens were considered more useful than timed collections, and, because of the effects of activity on albumin excretion rate, first-pass specimens on rising ('early morning urine') the most desirable. As urine concentration varies considerably between and within individuals, the general recommendation to measure an albumin:creatinine ratio was accepted, but if this was not organisationally practical a specific and sensitive concentration test could be used. Once positive, confirmation is recommended given the variability of albumin excretion rate from day to day. It was not felt that confirmation required a further clinic visit if one was already scheduled at three to four month intervals, unless there was evidence of renal impairment or non-diabetic renal disease. It seems sensible to measure serum creatinine annually at the same time. There is a need to consider the possibility of renal disease unrelated to diabetes.

Effectiveness and cost-effectiveness evidence suggests that ACE inhibitors should be used as first-line therapy in people with Type 1 diabetes once albumin excretion rate is detectably abnormal. Discussion of side effects noted the more serious of these (hyperkalaemia and acute renal impairment) related mostly to people with Type 2 diabetes. No direct evidence for angiotensin 2 receptor antagonists in Type 1 diabetes had been found, but as the microvascular complications of diabetes seem independent of aetiology of diabetes, the Group felt that evidence from Type 2 diabetes could be extrapolated. However, being more expensive, these should be reserved as second-line therapy. Combination therapy seems likely to be effective but no recommendation is appropriate until more evidence on benefit and risk in this area is available.

While it was not found that a low protein diet was sufficiently well supported to be recommended for people with evidence of established diabetic nephropathy, it was felt that formal advice on a non-high protein diet should be given. In the absence of useful evidence, the group were unable to set an arbitrary referral cut-off based on one biochemical measure, but agreed to leave this to local collaborative arrangements between specialists.

RECOMMENDATIONS

See also recommendations for blood pressure in section 8.3.

R112   All adults with Type 1 diabetes, with or without detected nephropathy, should be   D
       asked to bring in a first-pass morning urine specimen once a year. This should be
       sent for estimation of albumin:creatinine ratio. Estimation of urine albumin
       concentration alone is a poor alternative. Serum creatinine should be measured at
       the same time.

R113   If an abnormal surveillance result is obtained (in the absence of proteinuria/urinary   DS
       tract infection), the test should be repeated at each clinic visit or at least every
       three to four months, and the result taken as confirmed if a further specimen (out
       of two more) is also abnormal (>2.5 mg/mmol for men, >3.5 mg/mmol for women).

R114   Other renal disease should be suspected: DS
       - in the absence of progressive retinopathy
       - if blood pressure is particularly high
       - if proteinuria develops suddenly
       - if significant haematuria is present
       - in the presence of systemic ill health.

R115   The significance of a finding of abnormal albumin excretion rate should be discussed   D
       with the person concerned.

R116   ACE inhibitors should be started and (with usual precautions) titrated to full dose in   A
       all adults with confirmed nephropathy (including those with microalbuminuria alone)
       and Type 1 diabetes.

R117   If ACE inhibitors are not tolerated, angiotensin 2 receptor antagonists should be   B
       substituted. Combination therapy is not recommended at present.

R118   Blood pressure should be maintained below 130/80 mmHg by addition of other   D
       anti-hypertensive drugs if necessary.

R119   Adults with Type 1 diabetes and nephropathy should be advised about the advantages   B
       of not following a high protein diet.

R120   Referral criteria for tertiary care should be agreed between local diabetes specialists   D
       and nephrologists.

11 | Management of late complications: diabetes foot problems

11.1 Screening and surveillance of diabetic foot problems

▷ Rationale

Foot ulceration, foot infection, foot and limb amputation and some forms of deformity (including Charcot arthropathy) are major forms of disability arising from Type 1 diabetes. Prevention and management of such problems depends on detection of risk factors, and of markers of predisposing problems including neuropathy and vascular disease, as well as more diverse factors such as poor footwear and skin condition. Accurate and programmed surveillance for such risk factors is required if efficient use is to be made of education programmes and the services of those with special expertise in management of individuals with particularly high risk of foot ulceration.

▷ Evidence statements

Monitoring

The major risk factors for foot complications have been identified in several systematic reviews[174,244] as history of ulceration and lack of sensation.

The NICE *Clinical guidelines for Type 2 diabetes*[244] reported inconsistent evidence of markers associated with foot complications from nine studies using a range of methods and patient data. These included: old age, duration of diabetes, neuropathy, peripheral vascular disease, renal disease, foot deformities, plantar callus, previous ulceration or amputation, poor vision, poor footwear, cigarette smoking, social deprivation and social isolation (**NICE**).

The NICE guideline[244] also reported five surveys investigating additional risk factors for the elderly, concluded that suboptimal supervision of elderly patients in hospital, residential care and general practice increases their risk of ulceration and amputation (**NICE**).

Organisation of screening programmes

The SIGN guidelines[174] note that absence of reliable symptoms and the high prevalence of asymptomatic disease make foot screening essential (**IV**).

One large comparative trial in a systematic review[245] of a combined screening and foot protection programme reported a statistically significant reduction in major amputations over a two-year period compared to normal organisation of care (**Ia**).

The NICE clinical guidelines[244] report a Cochrane review comparing trials of general practice *vs* hospital care for recall and review of foot problems, and conclude that despite the methodological flaws in these trials a system of shared care – joint participation between hospitals and general practices – provides levels of surveillance as good as hospital diabetic clinic attendance alone (**NICE**).

Information exchange between specialists is advocated in one review in the NICE Type 2 diabetes guidelines.[244] However, no evidence exists to specify the components of these procedures (**NICE**).

The guidelines foot care working party[244] also endorsed the findings of Diabetes UK that a multidisciplinary team of professionals should be available to promptly provide the full range of appropriate foot care services to patients (**NICE**).

Detection of loss of foot sensation

SIGN guidelines[174] concluded from three studies that neuropathy screening performed by using clinical neuropathy disability scores, 10 g monofilaments or vibration perception thresholds, alone or in combination, have benefits in selecting patients at increased risk of foot ulceration (**DS**).

Additional techniques available for assessing neuropathic deficit that are considered in SIGN guidelines[174] include tactile circumferential discriminator, the graduated tuning fork, thermal discrimination devices and others. These techniques have not been prospectively evaluated but generally compare with other techniques for detection of ulcers (**IV**).

There is general agreement in systematic reviews and guidelines[174,244] that the 5.07 monofilament (10 g) is cheap and easy to use compared to other neuropathic tests and is the recommended screening test for neuropathy as a risk factor for diabetes foot ulcers (**IV/NICE**).

A systematic review[246] of a particular monofilament and other threshold tests for preventing ulceration and amputation in people with diabetes found this design of monofilament correlated best with the presence or history of an ulcer. Evidence varies as to the appropriate number of sites to use with this technique, the majority of studies testing at ≥1 site. The plantar surface of the forefoot provides the best discrimination between those who did and did not have ulcers (**III**).

Four prospective studies included in a systematic review[246] described a strong predictive ability of the monofilament test for future foot ulceration and amputation and a high reproducibility (**DS**).

Within a systematic review[246] two non-randomised studies reported physical symptoms of tingling, burning, hyperaesthesia and other uncomfortable sensations affecting >40% of people with diabetes after diagnosis. However, two separate studies reported poor correlation of pain symptoms with foot ulceration (**III**).

Prospective evidence is sparse for traditional clinical assessment,[246] using pinprick, tuning fork vibration or light touch with a cotton wisp. While the reproducibility of these investigations is low, replicability is slightly better for ankle jerks; however these tests are considered poor predictors of ulceration (**DS**).

Two-point discrimination was shown in one study in a well-produced systematic review[246] to be more sensitive but less specific than monofilament or vibration perception threshold (VPT) testing. Temperature sensation was found in two studies to be cumbersome and irritating and correlated less well with risk of ulceration compared to monofilament or VPT (**DS**).

One further medium-sized diagnostic study[247] described the comparability of a new technique combining a monofilament and pinprick test to reference standard tests. The new technique was found to have good correlation with VPT and a neuropathy disability score assessment, and a specificity and sensitivity of roughly 80% and 70% respectively in detecting both neuropathy disability score and VPT results identifying moderate to severe neuropathy (**DS**).

Detection of peripheral vascular disease

Screening for vascular insufficiency is less well documented than ulceration in existing reviews[174] (**IV**).

Two studies in the SIGN guidelines[174] note that absence of pedal pulses can be used in first-line screening as a guide to peripheral vascular disease. Evidence from one study urges caution when evaluating ankle pressure and pressure indices, which can be falsely elevated in people with diabetes (**DS**).

A systematic review[248] of observational studies noted a restricted accuracy of pedal pulses in identifying severe peripheral ischaemia (**DS**).

The validity of Doppler ultrasonography to determine ankle-branchial index as an indicator of peripheral blood flow was also questioned by one study in a systematic review.[248] The study noted that calcification of the media of the distal arteries, common in diabetes, may lead to artificially high systolic pressure in the ankle (**DS**).

▷ Health economic evidence

The health economic search found no papers specific to foot care screening or treatment in Type 1 diabetes. As the Type 2 diabetes foot care guideline will use all the information identified in the health economic searches, and may use other information excluded in the search process, the specific health economic recommendations from this guideline should be applied here.

The only exception to this comes in the cost-effectiveness of cultured human dermis where additional modelling was undertaken. Two economic evaluations[376–7] were identified from the literature for Dermagraft, of which one paper used UK cost data,[377] but the results were unpublished. The remaining paper[376] considers French cost-effectiveness in terms of cost per ulcer healed over 52 weeks. This model was replicated by the health economist in the GDG, but its findings could not be duplicated. No conclusion can therefore be drawn from these studies.

This replicated model was used to construct an estimate of the cost-effectiveness of Dermagraft in QALY terms using published health utility values. Dermagraft does not appear to be a cost-effective treatment for diabetic foot ulcers on the basis of this model. Furthermore, as the clinical data underlying this model relates to long-standing ulcers that may be less likely to heal with standard treatment, the general cost-effectiveness of Dermagraft for all non-recurrent ulcers free of infection is likely to be worse than the figures produced here.

▷ Consideration

The group noted that this area had been examined by other quality guideline groups both internationally and for Type 2 diabetes. No reason for being inconsistent with those recommendations could be found, although for the most part people with foot problems and Type 1 diabetes had predominantly neuropathic problems rather than neuroischaemic problems. Annual foot review was thought desirable for reasons of both foot surveillance and education. The simple and effective utility of the monofilament was noted.

RECOMMENDATIONS

R121   Structured foot surveillance should be at one-year intervals, and should include   D
        educational assessment and education input commensurate with the assessed risk.

R122   The reasons for, and success of, foot surveillance systems should be properly conveyed   D
        to adults with Type 1 diabetes, so that attendance is not reduced by ignorance of need.

R123   Inspection and examination of feet should include: D
        ● skin condition
        ● shape and deformity
        ● shoes
        ● impaired sensory nerve function
        ● vascular supply (including peripheral pulses).

R124   Use of a 10 g monofilament plus non-traumatic pin prick is advised for detection of   DS
        impairment of sensory nerve function sufficient to significantly raise risk of foot
        ulceration.

11.2   Management of foot ulceration and associated risk factors

▷   Rationale

Diabetes foot problems lead to significant morbidity and healthcare costs from foot ulceration and limb amputation. In Type 1 diabetes the predominant risk factor is the development of somatic sensory neuropathy, although peripheral vascular disease may contribute to the risks in some people. Poor blood glucose control can interfere with healing and control of infection where skin damage occurs.

▷   Evidence statements

There were no randomised controlled trials identified from the search of interventions for managing foot ulceration and infection in populations with Type 1 diabetes specifically. We therefore recommend following the Type 2 diabetes guideline for foot care, which considered evidence from trials with populations with Type 2 diabetes, and mixed Type 1 and Type 2 diabetes (**www.nice.org.uk**) (**NICE**).

▷   Consideration

The group noted the draft recommendations of the updated Type 2 diabetes foot care guideline, and the differences between Type 1 and Type 2 diabetes in respect of this area, mainly arising as a result of the lesser impact of peripheral vascular disease in people with Type 1 diabetes. The importance of trained foot care personnel was noted from the evidence statements in chapter 5. Disappointingly there was little evidence on the effectiveness of the different antibiotic regimens employed. The sometimes rapid progression from the start of ulceration to cellulitis was felt to justify very rapid referral and review by a specialist team where ulceration is detected.

The economic analysis provided to the group was felt to be secure in suggesting that human cultured dermis was not a cost-effective option in the context of the current NHS.

At the time of review by the group the evidence on Charcot osteoarthropathy management was felt to be incomplete, and the group did not reach any conclusions on the subject. A recommendation was based on the draft of the updated NICE guideline on foot care in Type 2 diabetes.

RECOMMENDATIONS

Foot complication surveillance

R125   On the basis of findings from foot care surveillance, foot ulceration risk should be   D
        categorised into:
- low current risk (normal sensation and palpable pulses)
- increased risk (impaired sensory nerve function or absent pulses, or other risk factor)
- high risk (impaired sensory nerve function and absent pulses or deformity or skin changes, or previous ulcer)
- ulcer present.

Foot care management

R126   For people found to be at increased risk or high risk of foot complications: B
- arrange specific assessment of other contributory risk factors including deformity, smoking, level of blood glucose control
- arrange/reinforce specific foot care education, and review those at high risk as part of a formal foot ulcer prevention programme
- consider the provision of special footwear, including insoles and orthoses, if there is a deformity, callosities or previous ulcer.

R127   For people with an ulcerated foot: B
- arrange referral to a specialist diabetes foot care team incorporating specifically-trained foot care specialists (usually state-registered podiatrists) within one to two days if there is no overt infection of the ulcer or surrounding tissues, or as an emergency if such infection is present
- use antibiotics if there is any evidence of infection of the ulcer or surrounding tissues, and continue these long-term if infection is recurrent
- use foot dressings taking account of cost according to local experience, ensuring arrangements are in place to monitor and change dressings frequently (often daily) accordingly to need
- remove dead tissue from diabetic foot ulcers
- consider the use of off-loading techniques (such as contact casting) for people with neuropathic foot ulcers
- do not use cultured human dermis (or equivalent), hyperbaric oxygen therapy, topical ketanserin or growth factors in routine foot ulcer management
- consider ensuring complete and effective foot education through the use of graphic visualisations of the consequences of ill-managed foot ulceration in people with recurrent ulceration or previous amputation
- review progress in ulcer healing frequently (daily to monthly) according to need
- if peripheral vascular disease is detected, refer for early assessment by a specialist vascular team.

Charcot osteoarthropathy

R128   Adults with suspected or diagnosed Charcot osteoarthropathy should be referred   **D**
immediately to a multidisciplinary diabetes foot care team.

12 | Management of late complications: diabetes nerve damage

12.1 Diagnosis and management of erectile dysfunction

▷ Rationale

Erectile dysfunction in men with diabetes is common, and to a greater extent than in the matched general population. There is some debate as to whether professionals should actively ask about erectile problems on a recurrent basis (perhaps yearly), or only respond to self-reported problems. There have been dramatic changes in the approach to male erectile dysfunction in recent years, stimulated by the advent of the phosphodiesterase type 5 (PDE5) inhibitors.

▷ Evidence statements

Significance of patient-reported sexual symptomatology in predicting actual physiological measures of sexual dysfunction

A medium-sized cross-sectional cohort study[249] in people with diabetes mellitus evaluated the significance of patient-reported sexual symptomatology in predicting penile tip and base rigidity, tip and base duration of erectile episode. This study reports that the presence of morning erections was associated with increased Rigiscan values of tip rigidity (r=0.64), base rigidity (r=0.58), tip duration of erectile episode (r=0.65) and base duration of erectile episodes (r=0.57), all demonstrating significant relationships (**IIa**).

Reports of fuller erectile quality were also significantly associated with increased Rigiscan values of tip rigidity (r=0.58), base rigidity (r=0.42), tip duration of erectile episode (r=0.67) and base duration of erectile episode (r=0.71).[249] Other significant associations found in this cohort study included intact ejaculatory capacity being associated with increased Rigiscan measures of tip rigidity (r=0.45). Tip duration of erectile episode (r=0.56) and base duration of erectile episode (r=0.30) were also related to Rigiscan measures in the same study.[249]

A significant inverse relationship was found between symptom frequency and the Rigiscan measure of base duration of erectile episodes, with greater symptom frequency being associated with diminished duration values of erectile episodes at the penile base (r=-0.39)[249] (**IIa**).

Correlations of lower limb nerve fibre abnormalities with erectile dysfunction

A medium-sized cross-sectional cohort study[250] aimed to characterise the neuropathy in erectile dysfunction, as well as to identify nerve fibre subtypes that may be preferentially affected. Patients were evaluated with a symptom questionnaire based on the Michigan Neuropathy Screening instrument questionnaire and examined clinically. Sural and peroneal nerve-conduction studies and quantitative sensory and autonomic tests (using the staging system of Dyck) were used to detect nerve abnormalities in the lower limbs. Various methodological limitations inherent to the study limited the validity of the results derived from the trial (**IIa**).

Relationship of symptoms of depression, sexual dysfunction and neuropathy in women

A small cross-sectional cohort study[251] assessed the relationship between symptoms of depression (as measured by the Beck Depression Inventory and the Hamilton Psychiatric Rating Scale), sexual dysfunction (as measured by a questionnaire which asked patients to rate their symptoms on a scale from 0 to 10), and neuropathy (as measured by the visual analogue scale). However, various methodological limitations inherent to the study limit the validity of the results derived from the trial, and should not be used as the basis for a positive recommendation (**IIa**).

Sildenafil

One large multicentre study of sildenafil at 100 mg/day compared to placebo in men with erectile dysfunction and Type 1 or Type 2 diabetes[252] found significantly more men were able to achieve and to maintain erections with sildenafil than placebo at 12 weeks. Another 11 outcomes from questionnaire-based evaluation of male sexual function described significant improvement with the intervention drug, however there were no differences in indices of frequency and level of sexual desire. Erectile function was improved regardless of age, duration of erectile dysfunction, duration of diabetes or type of diabetes, and the incidence of adverse arterial events was similar in both groups (**Ib**).

A smaller prospective study from the UK[253] found that sildenafil at 25 mg or 50 mg, compared to placebo, significantly improved adjusted duration of penile rigidity at base and tip. In addition, there was an improved number of erections hard enough for sexual intercourse with either dose, with no serious adverse events being related to treatment (**Ib**).

▷ Consideration

The group noted the problems surrounding asking all men about impotence, but suggested a reasonable approach to this problem is to enquire as to whether individuals were 'troubled by sexual dysfunction'. It was not felt that the current opportunities for assisting women with problems of organic sexual dysfunction secondary to diabetes could justify routine enquiry. The group noted the licensing in 2003 of two additional PDE5 inhibitors to sildenafil, and felt that the lack of comparative trials meant that any recommendations should be for the drug class rather than any individual agent. Men still having a problem after a trial of PDE5 inhibitors had failed might have their needs met by expertise available in a variety of care situations, suggesting that the site of such care and advice could not be specified.

RECOMMENDATIONS

R129   Men should be asked annually whether erectile dysfunction is an issue.   **D**

R130   A PDE5 (phosphodiesterase-5) inhibitor drug, if not contraindicated, should be offered   **A**
where erectile dysfunction is a problem.

R131   Referral to a service offering other medical and surgical management of erectile   **D**
dysfunction should be discussed where PDE5 inhibitors are not successful.

12.2   Diagnosis and management of autonomic neuropathy

▷   Rationale

Autonomic neuropathy is a late complication of diabetes that presents in diverse ways and affects a variety of organ symptoms including the skin (sweating), blood vessels (orthostatic hypotension), gastrointestinal tract (gastroparesis, diarrhoea), heart (cardiac arrest), bladder and sexual function. It may blunt the symptoms of hypoglycaemia. Considerable morbidity occurs as a result of many of these problems.

▷   Evidence statements

Progression of autonomic neuropathy

A long-term follow-up study measured the progression of symptoms of autonomic neuropathy in 76 people with Type 1 diabetes and over nine years.[254] This study found that of all the symptoms of autonomic neuropathy only gastroparesis was found to have increased in prevalence from baseline. At nine years after entering the study the only other symptoms reported were diarrhoea, impotence, loss of vaginal lubrication, hypoglycaemia unawareness and postural hypotension, and these were reported in not more than 9% of the study sample. There was a tendency for many symptoms such as hypoglycaemia unawareness to recover with time (III).

Symptoms of autonomic neuropathy

Two descriptive reviews were located that suggested possible symptoms due to autonomic neuropathy across diabetes populations. One review[255] suggested impotence, unexplained diarrhoea, faecal incontinence, unexplained urinary symptoms (increased period between micturition, muted sensation of bladder fullness, frequency, urinary incontinence, unexplained bladder dilation), postural dizziness or faintness, gustatory sweating, dry feet, unexplained bloating, early satiety, fullness, nausea, vomiting, unexplained dysphagia and unexplained ankle oedema. The authors suggested that tests for autonomic neuropathy may help in defining neuropathic aetiology. Another review[256] found that autonomic symptoms can be vague and may present insidiously, and that nerve damage can be found in people without symptoms being manifest. It is suggested that a mixed presentation is usual with a combination of postural hypotension, nocturnal diarrhoea, gastric problems, bladder symptoms, abnormal sweating, impotence or a failure to recognise that hypoglycaemia is likely. In addition people with severe symptoms may also have advanced retinopathy, nephropathy and somatic neuropathy (IV).

Aldose reductase inhibitors

Three randomised controlled trials have investigated the effect of ponalrestat on autonomic nerve function in mixed diabetes cohorts. Two small and short-term studies found no benefit of ponalrestat over placebo in terms of heart rate variability[257] or standard tests of autonomic function,[258] although a vibration perception measure or peripheral neuropathy did show a significant improvement with the intervention drug after 16 weeks of therapy.[257] However the potential methodological limitations of this study would not recommend it for the basis for recommendations (**Ib**).

A larger multicentre trial[259] also testing the effect of 600 mg of ponalrestat compared to placebo found heart rate response to standing was significantly greater on the intervention drug while HbA$_{1c}$ remained constant throughout the period, and with no effect on frequency of adverse events, although only a third of the study population displayed abnormal autonomic neuropathy from tests, with the sample being drawn from people with diabetes and peripheral neuropathy (**Ib**).

A long-term study[260] found that there was a significant increase in indices of postural index and heart rate variability after two years of treatment with tolrestat compared with placebo, with changes in autonomic function not being influenced by changes in HbA$_{1c}$ level. This study was conducted in people with diabetes who displayed abnormalities in two or more standard autonomic function tests and used a dose of 200 mg/day tolrestat (**Ib**).

ACE inhibitors

Two small studies with medium-term follow-up investigated the potential of the angiotensin converting enzyme inhibitor quinapril to improve the heart rate variability of people with diabetic autonomic neuropathy. One study[261] found total heart power (by 24-hour ECG) to be improved with quinapril compared to placebo as was high frequency power at six months. In addition there was a significant increase in the level of heart rate variability at both three and six months. A similar study for 12 months[262] found quinapril to have beneficial effects on all heart rate frequency domains, and the low frequency to high frequency power ratio to be lower (improved) with quinapril than placebo, and this held for analysis of morning, evening, or night-time comparisons. The study also found quinapril to reduce heart rate to 12 months although no effect was seen on blood pressure. No complications of diabetic autonomic neuropathy or hospitalisations were reported (**Ib**).

No studies were identified that determined the effects of quinapril on symptoms of autonomic neuropathy.

Indirect cholinergic agent cisapride

A small crossover trial of 20 mg cisapride compared to placebo in a mixed diabetes population[263] found no increase in antral or duodenal motility with the intervention drug; however, antral-duodenal coordination was significantly improved when fasting, and at other meals (**Ib**).

Erythromycin

Three small crossover trials of erythromycin compared to placebo in people with Type 1 diabetes and documented gastroparesis found short-term improvement in emptying of solids and mixed results with liquids with oral[264,265] or intravenous[266] administration, without side effects. However no improvements in symptoms scores were reported and larger scale and longer trials will be required to prove efficacy (**Ib**).

▷ Health economic evidence

No health economic papers were found regarding the diagnosis of either autonomic neuropathy or gastroparesis. One paper[378] was identified in the cost-effectiveness of management for painful neuropathy. However, as a review of other evidence, specific cost-effectiveness data was limited to recommending intensive treatment to reduce complications.

▷ Consideration

The group noted that the manifestations of autonomic neuropathy often occurred independently of each other, with very significant overlap into many other super-specialties of medicine (for example dermatology, gastroenterology, urology). Accordingly, the topic addressed a wider range of diagnostic and management issues than could be tackled in a diabetes guideline. Nevertheless the importance of alertness to, and detection of, these conditions was clearly relevant to the practice of the diabetes team. Of specific relevance is gastroparesis because of the effect of this condition on blood glucose control, but the group recognised that the diagnosis of this condition was not easy or reliable, and the treatments available only partially and erratically successful.

RECOMMENDATIONS

R132	In adults with Type 1 diabetes on insulin therapy who have erratic blood glucose control (or unexplained bloating or vomiting), the diagnosis of gastroparesis should be considered.	D
R133	In adults with Type 1 diabetes who have altered perception of hypoglycaemia the possibility of sympathetic nervous system damage as a contributory factor should be considered.	D
R134	In adults with Type 1 diabetes who have unexplained diarrhoea, particularly at night, the possibility of autonomic neuropathy affecting the gut should be considered.	D
R135	Care should be taken when prescribing antihypertensive drugs not to expose people to the risks of orthostatic hypotension as a result of the combined effects of sympathetic autonomic neuropathy and blood pressure lowering drugs.	D
R136	Adults with Type 1 diabetes who have bladder emptying problems should be investigated for the possibility of autonomic neuropathy affecting the bladder, unless other explanations are adequate.	D

R137   The management of the symptoms of autonomic neuropathy should include standard   D
interventions for the manifestations encountered (for example, for erectile dysfunction
or abnormal sweating).

R138   For adults with Type 1 diabetes with diagnosed or suspected gastroparesis a trial   D
of prokinetic drugs is indicated (metoclopramide or domperidone, with cisapride as
third line if necessary).

Anaesthesia and autonomic neuropathy

R139   Anaesthetists should be aware of the possibility of parasympathetic autonomic   D
neuropathy affecting the heart in adults with Type 1 diabetes who are listed for
procedures under general anaesthetic and who have evidence of somatic neuropathy
or other manifestations of autonomic neuropathy.

12.3   Optimum management of painful neuropathy

▷   Rationale

Symptomatic neuropathy is unusual amongst the forms of diabetes tissue damage in that it is a
relatively early manifestation of the effects of hyperglycaemia, which may go into remission
with progression of nerve damage (nerve death) or recovery of nerve fibre function. The
symptoms are protean in nature, and often very troublesome to the person with diabetes,
especially if sleep is disturbed. Management can be difficult.

▷   Evidence statements

Anticonvulsants

One large meta-analysis[267] found a significant benefit of at least 50% pain relief with people
with anticonvulsants compared to placebo. The relative risk estimates showed that anticonvulsants had a significantly increased incidence of adverse effects compared with placebo for
minor but not major harm (**Ia**).

One small, randomised controlled trial of gabapentin[268] found an improvement over placebo
control on a pain questionnaire at 12 weeks but with no significant improvement on a visual
analogue pain scale, or present pain intensity. No significant adverse events were reported in
either study arm but minor events drowsiness, fatigue and imbalance were more common in
the population on gabapentin than on placebo (**Ib**).

The differences in mean pain intensities between the intervention and control groups were
significant after eight weeks at lamotrigine doses of 200, 300 and 400 mg in a small-scale
prospective randomised trial.[269] This study found no significant changes in assessment of
McGill Pain Questionnaire, Beck Depression Inventory and Pain Disability Index (**Ib**).

Antidepressants

One large meta-analysis found a significant benefit of at least 50% pain relief with people with
antidepressants compared to placebo[267] with pooled analyses of tricyclic antidepressants
showing significant benefit but no benefit with selective serotonin re-uptake inhibitors.

Tricyclic antidepressants used were prescribed in doses in the low to moderate range for depression. Antidepressants had a significantly increased incidence of adverse effects compared with placebo with typical antimuscarinic effects of dry mouth, constipation and blurred vision. Also major events (leading to withdrawal from the trial) were more common with antidepressants than placebo, the number needed to harm (NNH) for a major adverse effect with antidepressants compared with placebo was 17 (**Ia**).

A small short-term randomised controlled trial[270] investigating mean pain intensity diary scores in a six-week within-patient comparison, showed that desipramine was superior to placebo. No significant difference between incidence of adverse events or withdrawals between desipramine and placebo groups (**Ib**).

Other therapies

Amantadine: A small randomised controlled trial with a one-week follow-up[271] found amantadine infusion at 200 mg in 500 ml 0.9% saline infusion over three-hour period caused a significant clinically relevant reduction in pain score when compared with placebo, and caused a significant improvement in the neuropathy symptom score. Following amantadine, there was a clinically significant subjective tenfold improvement in pain relief (**Ib**).

Capsaicin: A meta-analysis[272] comparing a range of studies with outcomes from four to eight weeks found capsaicin cream produced significantly higher response rates than placebo cream for physician assessment of global pain in two of the trials, but not in the other two (**Ia**).

Clonidine: No statistically significant difference between intervention and control groups in patients' pain record diary or pain intensity levels in two randomised trials of clonidine.[273,274] In the patients completing the study, dry mouth and drowsiness tended to occur more commonly with clonidine than placebo[273] (**Ib**).

Gamma-linolenic acid: Compared with placebo, dietary supplementation with gamma-linolenic acid was reported as being associated with significant clinical, neuropsychological and quantitative sensory improvement in established distal diabetic polyneuropathy in the medium term.[275] A significant improvement in the gamma-linolenic acid group compared with the placebo group was seen in nine variables: symptom scores, median MCV (m/s), peroneal MCV (m/s), median CMAP (mV), peroneal CMAP (mV), median SNAP (μV), sural SNAP (μV), ankle HT (°C), wrist HT (°C). This study recruited only people with Type 2 diabetes (**Ib**).

A second trial[276] confirms this with gamma-linolenic acid being significantly superior in improving neuropsychological, neurological and thermal sensation parameters of diabetic neuropathy compared with placebo over a one-year period. A significant improvement in the gamma-linolenic acid group compared with the placebo group was seen in: peroneal MNCV, median MNCV, extensor digitorium brevis CMAP, thenar CMAP, sural SNAP, median SNAP, wrist heat threshold, wrist cold threshold, arm muscle strength, arm tendon reflexes, leg tendon reflexes, arm sensation, leg sensation. Subgroup analysis showed improvement of outcome parameters with the gamma-linolenic acid was greater in patients with initial HbA_{1c} <10% than those with HbA_{1c} >10% (**Ib**).

Isosorbide dinitrate (ISDN): A small crossover trial[277] showed significant reductions in pain and burning sensation using the ISDN spray compared with placebo. During the ISDN phase of the study, two patients developed mild transient headaches, which resolved spontaneously and did not affect overall adherence with the spray (**Ib**).

Mexiletine: Trials of mexiletine have provided mixed results in terms of efficacy for pain reduction in people with diabetes and painful neuropathy. This difference in effect could be due to clinical differences in study populations, doses utilised or length of follow-up measured (**Ib**).

A significant reduction in pain during night-time (as estimated by the visual analogue scale score for pain) was observed in the mexiletine 675 mg group compared with the placebo group as was a significant reduction in sleep disturbances in a large multicentre randomised trial.[278] No significant difference between groups in daytime pain or global assessment of efficacy was recorded. However, another study[279] showed no improvement in the McGill Questionnaire or on the visual analogue scale for pain to five weeks (**Ib**).

In contrast a study of mexiletine compared to placebo for 26 weeks[280] found that the Five Item Symptom Scale Score was improved in all but one patient during treatment with mexiletine, but in only two patients during the placebo phase. Mexiletine significantly improved pain, dysaesthesia and paraesthesia. During treatment with mexiletine the visual analogue score fell significantly. Three patients had mild side effects when treated with mexiletine, including nausea, hiccough and tremor (**Ib**).

Tramadol: A medium-scaled prospective randomised trial[281] of tramadol at up to 200 mg/day found that by day 14 people in the tramadol group had less pain than patients in the placebo group. This benefit lasted through to the end of the trial at day 42. They also scored better on outcomes of physical and social functioning. No statistically significant differences between treatments were noted for current health perception, psychological distress, overall role functioning and the two overall sleep problem indexes and sleep subscales. The most common adverse events in the tramadol group were nausea (23%), constipation (22%), headache (17%) and somnolence (12%). Nine patients treated with tramadol and one treated with placebo discontinued due to adverse events. The most common adverse events leading to discontinuation of tramadol were nausea and dyspepsia. However, this study recruited only people with Type 2 diabetes (**Ib**).

▷ Consideration

The group noted that the severity of neuropathic symptoms varied considerably between individuals. Many of the well-established drugs were used outside licensed indications in contrast to the newest drugs. Established clinical practice, as in most areas of pain control, uses a stepped approach, and no reason for challenging that was found. Nevertheless, the group was also aware that prescribing habits and long review intervals could lead to suboptimal management where therapies proved ineffective, both through a failure to recognise an unsuccessful trial of therapy and through over-slow dose titration. In the absence of comparative studies, while gabapentin was believed more effective than tricyclic drugs, the need for dose titration and problems of intolerance together with cost suggested the older drugs to be worth a trial first. Other drugs were now felt by the group to be reserved for people failing trials of tricyclic drugs and gabapentin. The group were aware of difficulties with evidence on gamma-linolenic acid, which meant that it could not be considered further for this guideline. The group also noted the availability of local pain management teams for people whose pain does not respond to conventional measures.

RECOMMENDATIONS

R140	Use of simple analgesics (paracetamol, aspirin) and local measures (bed cradles) are recommended as a first step, but if trials of these measures are ineffective, they should be discontinued and other measures should be tried.	D
R141	Where initial measures fail, a low to medium dose of a tricyclic drug should be used, timed to be taken before the time of day the symptoms are troublesome; adults with Type 1 diabetes should be advised that this is a trial of therapy.	A
R142	Where an adequate trial of tricyclic drugs fails, a trial of gabapentin should be started, and not stopped unless ineffective at the maximum tolerated dose or at least 1,800 mg per day.	A
R143	If treatment with gabapentin is unsuccessful, carbamazepine and phenytoin should be considered.	D
R144	Where severe chronic pain persists despite trials of other measures, opiate analgesia may be considered. At this stage the assistance of the local chronic pain management service should be sought.	D
R145	Professionals should be alert to the psychological consequences of chronic painful neuropathy, and offer appropriate management where they are identified.	D
R146	Where drug therapy is successful in alleviating symptoms, trials of reduced dosage and cessation of therapy should be considered after six months of treatment.	D

R147   Where neuropathic symptoms cannot be adequately controlled it is useful, to help   D
individuals cope, to explain:

- the reasons for the problem
- the likelihood of remission in the medium term
- the role of improved blood glucose control.

13 | Management of special situations

13.1 Adults who are newly diagnosed

▷ Rationale

The time following diagnosis is one of marked stress for many adults with diabetes. However, decisions taken at this time may have a long-term impact, and to be accurate and effective would appear to need fairly complete assessment of medical and lifestyle factors. These can be expected to affect choice of therapy and monitoring requirements, educational requirements, input from different members of the multidisciplinary team, site of care and the need for involvement of other health-related services and perhaps employers and other institutions.

▷ Evidence statements

Organisation of initial assessment planning

Consensus in the ADA guidelines[76] suggests that medical evaluation is made to classify the person presenting as a basis for a management plan and to assess complications. This is echoed by Diabetes UK recommendations for management in primary care[282] which indicate that a planned programme of diabetes care should include systems for ensuring assessment and acute management of all newly-diagnosed patients. In addition, American guidelines from the Department of Veterans Affairs[283] identify initial assessment as a useful tool to review systems and set priorities for care (**IV**).

Content of the initial assessment plan

All of the guidelines reviewed are aimed at a mixed diabetic population and do not specify any specific features of initial assessment that are particular to people with Type 1 diabetes. All guidance suggests that assessment should look for co-morbid conditions that people with diabetes are more commonly at risk from[282–5] and should consider factors that may affect the management of diabetes such as COPD, substance misuse and depression.[283–5] Factors that may precipitate diabetes secondary to other medical conditions should also be considered[283] (**IV**).

Other factors of initial assessment that can aid management planning that are widely suggested included physical examinations, laboratory tests including lipid profile, urinalysis and ECG.[282–3,285] Consideration for referral is advised for (**IV**):

- urgent hospitalisation if patient is clearly unwell,[282] or
- where specialist examination is required for eye exam, family planning, diabetes education, behavioural advice or foot disorders.[285]

Consistent documentation of assessment is widely recommended,[282–3] and initial assessment should be used for the baseline of an individualised management plan[282,285] (**IV**).

Benefit of initial assessment plan

No interventional studies were identified that assess the affect on outcomes of improved initial assessment planning. It may be assumed that benefits may accrue in terms of understanding and satisfaction with care, and potentially with adherence to management plans, although these cannot be quantified at this time (**IV**).

▷ Health economic evidence

The health economic searches produced no studies giving guidance on appropriate insulin regimens for those newly diagnosed with Type 1 diabetes.

▷ Consideration

The group noted that this was not an area in which to expect RCT evidence of different styles of initial management planning, and endorsed in general the views expressed in other recent guidelines for people with Type 1 diabetes. An overlap with the education recommendations of this guideline (see 6.1) was noted.

RECOMMENDATIONS

R148   At the time of diagnosis (or if necessary after the management of critically   **D**
decompensated metabolism) the professional team should develop with, and explain to, the adult with Type 1 diabetes a plan for their early care. To agree such a plan will generally require:
- medical assessment to:
  - ensure security of diagnosis of type of diabetes
  - ensure appropriate acute care is given when needed
  - review and detect potentially confounding disease and drugs
  - detect adverse vascular risk factors
- environmental assessment to understand:
  - social, home, work and recreational circumstances of the individual and carers
  - their preferences in nutrition and physical activity
  - other relevant factors such as substance use
- cultural and educational assessment to identify prior knowledge and to enable optimal advice and planning about:
  - treatment modalities
  - diabetes education programmes
- assessment of emotional state to determine the appropriate pace of education.

The results of the assessment should be used to agree a future care plan.

R149   Elements of an individualised and culturally-appropriate plan will include: **D**
- sites and timescales of diabetes education including nutritional advice (see section 6.1, 'Education programmes for adults with Type 1 diabetes' and 6.3, 'Dietary management')
- initial treatment modalities (see section 7.3, 'Insulin regimens' and 7.4, 'Insulin delivery')
- means of self-monitoring (see section 6.2, 'Self-monitoring of glood glucose')

Table 6 Some items of the initial diabetes assessment	
● Acute medical history	● General examination
● Social, cultural and educational history/lifestyle review	● Weight/body mass index
	● Foot/eye/vision examination
● Complications history/symptoms	● Urine albumin excretion/urine protein/serum creatinine
● Long-term/recent diabetes history	
● Other medical history/systems	● Psychological well-being
● Family history of diabetes/arterial disease	● Attitudes to medicine and self-care
● Drug history/current drugs	● Immediate family and social relationships and availability of informal support
● Vascular risk factors	
● Smoking	

- means and frequency of communication with the professional team
- follow-up consultations including surveillance at annual review (see the chapters on the management of late complications (chapters 9 to 12))
- management of arterial risk factors (see chapter 8, 'Arterial risk control').

R150   After the initial plan is agreed, arrangements should be put in place to implement it   D
without inappropriate delay, and to provide for feedback and modification of the plan
over the ensuing weeks.

13.2   Diabetic ketoacidosis

▷   Rationale

The management of diabetic ketoacidosis (DKA) is a topic which has attracted considerable attention over 40 years, because it can carry a high fatality risk if suboptimally managed. If optimally managed, the fatality and morbidity rates are very low. The topic is not easily addressed within a general diabetes guideline, being large enough for a guideline of its own. The approach below is to address some broad principles and specific topics of contention, rather than present a detailed protocol.

▷   Evidence statements

Insulin therapy

Continuous *vs* intermittent insulin therapy for DKA was evaluated in one small randomised study.[286] Insulin was administered as bolus injections (50 U/2h) compared to continuous insulin infusion (10 U/h) and low dose continuous insulin infusion (2 U/h) with an initial loading dose. To reduce plasma glucose concentrations, continuous infusion is as effective as intermittent insulin therapy at 10 U/h, with reduction to 5 U/h when plasma glucose <300 mg/100 ml. DKA recovery rate was significantly reduced following the very low dose continuous infusion regimen (Ib).

Another small study[287] showed that low doses of insulin given by intermittent intramuscular (IM) injection or by constant intravenous (IV) infusion after an initial IV loading dose are similarly effective in controlling DKA. Time to recovery of DKA and total insulin dose required did not differ between the two treatment groups (**Ib**).

A comparison[288] of different possible routes of insulin delivery in treating DKA showed similar efficacy for IV, IM and subcutaneous (SC) administered insulin therapy. No significant differences were seen for the time to metabolic recovery or total insulin dose or fluid replacement requirements. Patients receiving IM insulin were most likely to require additional insulin loading dose to achieve an adequate initial response. In this report a significantly higher rate of decrease in glucose and ketone bodies was observed in the first two hours following IV insulin, but these differences were not maintained over the rest of the recovery period (**Ib**).

No significant differences in recovery rates were seen following the administration of human and porcine insulin for treatment of DKA in a prospective trial with a small study population of people with both Type 1 and Type 2 diabetes[289] (**Ib**).

Continuation of insulin administration past the usually cut-off point of near-normoglycaemia *vs* conventional insulin regimen (rehydration, electrolyte replacement and insulin at 5 U/h to near-normoglycaemia, that is blood glucose less than or equal to 10 mmol/l, and then at a reduced rate until clinical recovery) in one small study,[290] significantly increased the resolution of ketosis, measured as duration of elevated blood 3-hydroxybutyrate levels, and acidosis (**Ib**).

Bicarbonate therapy

Intravenous sodium bicarbonate therapy added to the treatment regimen for DKA was shown in a randomised trial with small sample size[291] to increase recovery of arterial pH and bicarbonate levels in the first two hours, but did not effect pCO_2 or blood glucose levels. All patients in the bicarbonate group developed hypokalaemia (**Ib**).

One study[292] compared the effect of two different intravenous bicarbonate doses (adjusted to initial arterial pH) on the recovery rate of DKA, with placebo. No significant differences were seen between the groups treated with bicarbonate or placebo (**Ib**).

In agreement with these studies, one small trial[293] showed intravenous bicarbonate therapy had no additional beneficial effect when compared to standard DKA therapy without bicarbonate supplementation (**IIa**).

No significant differences were seen after addition of phosphate therapy to treatment for DKA in a small trial.[294] A protective effect against hypophosphataemia was seen following phosphate treatment compared to placebo, but only on the first day of treatment (**Ib**).

An additional paper[295] also reported no evidence of clinical benefit of phosphate therapy compared to placebo (**Ib**).

Somatostatin therapy

One small study[296] concluded that addition of the somatostatin analogue octreotide to low-dose insulin therapy reduced the time taken for correction of ketonuria. However, no such effect was seen on recovery rate of hyperglycaemia and acidosis (**Ib**).

▷ Health economic evidence

The health economic searches found only one US-based costing study.[379] As such, no specific health economic guidance can be provided here.

▷ Consideration

DKA management was noted to be based on a mixture of types of evidence, pathological, pharmacokinetic, clinical outcomes, cohorts and trials.

It was noted that DKA management is:

- quite detailed
- often performed under the supervision of diverse groups of specialists
- dependent on careful monitoring if catastrophic outcome is to be avoided.

There was broad consensus on issues of management, which largely seem to revolve around ameliorating the acidosis and hyperglycaemia without inducing the possibly fatal complications of cerebral oedema, hypokalaemia or aspiration pneumonia. Moderation in speed and methods of correcting dehydration, hyperglycaemia and ketosis is combined with a high intensity of monitoring of the changing condition of the patient.

The group noted that there was no evidence at all for the use of bicarbonate in any situation, and that the consensus recommendations for its use below a pH of 6.9 were poorly grounded in either clinical experience or any kind of evidence.

The group noted that the nature of insulin pharmacokinetics and pharmacodynamics suggested that the detailed studies of ways of starting insulin infusions had no logical basis.

Clinical experience of management in adults suggested that acute respiratory distress syndrome ('fluid on the lung') was seen not infrequently in addition to cerebral oedema. While the evidence that either of these could be ameliorated by using lower rates of saline replacement was not good, nor was there any impression that in the non-shocked patients such lower rates were harmful. Accordingly they are recommended.

Members of the group had seen examples of glucose concentration escape after reaching near-normal glucose levels, and felt that the evidence-based lesson of the Belfast paper[290] (that these insulin-resistant patients require continued administration of higher rates of insulin than other patients on insulin infusions) was worth noting.

RECOMMENDATIONS

R151   Professionals managing DKA should be adequately trained including regular updating,   **D**
        and familiar with all aspects of its management which are associated with mortality and
        morbidity. These topics should include:
- fluid balance
- acidosis
- cerebral oedema
- electrolyte imbalance
- disturbed interpretation of familiar diagnostic tests (white cell count, body temperature, ECG)

- respiratory distress syndrome
- cardiac abnormalities
- precipitating causes
- infection management including opportunistic infections
- gastroparesis
- use of high dependency and intensive care units
- and the recommendations below.

Management of DKA should be in line with local clinical governance.

R152   Primary fluid replacement in DKA should be with isotonic saline, not given too rapidly   D
except in cases of circulatory collapse.

R153   Bicarbonate should not generally be used in the management of DKA.   A

R154   Intravenous insulin should be given by infusion in cases of DKA.   A

R155   In the management of DKA, once plasma glucose concentration has fallen to   D
10–15 mmol/l, glucose containing fluids should be given (not more than two litres in
24 hours) in combination with higher rates of insulin infusion than used in other
situations (for example 6 U/h – monitored for effect).

R156   Potassium replacement should begin early in DKA, with frequent monitoring for the   D
development of hypokalaemia.

R157   Phosphate replacement should not generally be used in the management of DKA.   A

R158   In patients whose conscious level is impaired, consideration should be given to   D
insertion of a nasogastric tube, urinary catheterisation to monitor urine production
and heparinisation.

R159   To reduce the risk of catastrophic outcomes in DKA, monitoring should be continuous   D
and review should cover all aspects of clinical management at frequent intervals.

13.3   Inpatient management

▷   Rationale

People with Type 1 diabetes often find that time in hospital, or other institutional care, is somewhat stressful. The delicate equilibrium they may have established with their insulin therapy can be destroyed by the change in routine, change in nutrition and the effects of illness and procedures. They find too often that the expertise they bring to their diabetes management is underused by staff with less knowledge of the condition than themselves. Special insulin regimens may be needed to cope with procedures which interfere with eating patterns, or which cause enough metabolic stress to otherwise disturb control of diabetes. In some acute situations there is evidence that special insulin management may improve the outcomes of other medical conditions.

The overwhelming majority of admissions of people with diabetes are for non-diabetes related medical and surgical conditions. Indeed the problems discussed above are likely to be greater when care is outside the responsibility of the multidisciplinary diabetes team. Accordingly the evidence search and recommendations are intended to cover hospital and other institutional care across all specialties. However, some aspects of continuing self-care will self-evidently not be relevant during extreme critical illness.

The principles espoused are seen as applying, in general, to other institutional care (prisons, residential and nursing homes) as well as hospital care.

▷ Evidence statements

Multidisciplinary team care

One study[297] showed a significant reduction in length of stay in hospital following supervision by a diabetes specialist nurse. Significant differences were also seen in patient satisfaction and diabetes knowledge, although not for readmission frequency, referral rates or quality of life (**Ib**).

A cohort study[298] showed a significant reduction in length of stay in medical and surgery wards in patients with diabetes following the introduction of a diabetes nurse advisor (**IIa**).

A prospective randomised study examining the impact of a specialist diabetes team on inpatient management[55] demonstrated a significant increase in documentation of instructions for blood glucose monitoring, insulin administration, received education and nutritional consultation. Patients were significantly less likely to be readmitted within three months following supervision by a specialist diabetes team (**Ia**).

Hospital procedures

A small prospective randomised trial of aggressive IV insulin therapy with glucose level checks every 15 to 30 minutes compared to standard insulin therapy in a mixed diabetes cohort undergoing cardiopulmonary bypass[299] found that phagocytic activity decreased less with the aggressive regimen at one hour post operation. There was no measurement of clinical outcomes in this trial (**Ib**).

A cohort study from the United States in a mixed diabetic population[300] found that blood glucose levels on the day of operation to the third post-operative day were significantly lower with continuous insulin infusion compared to individualised subcutaneous insulin injection. Also the risk of deep sternal wound infection following cardiac surgery was independently associated with receiving continuous insulin infusion in multivariate analysis (**IIa**).

In another trial including people with both Type 1 and Type 2 diabetes,[301] continuous IV infusion of insulin from an electrically-driven syringe produced no significant differences in plasma beta-hydroxybutyrate:acetoacetate ratio, lactate:pyruvate ratio or concentrations of cortisol and catecholamine compared with a two-hourly bolus IV insulin injection. The total amount of insulin and rate given was similar in both groups (**Ib**).

Two small studies of IV delivery of insulin compared to subcutaneous injection in either minor[302] or major[303] surgery found that median blood glucose can be reduced on the first postoperative day with IV delivery although this did not hold true for all time points at which levels were tested, and that more measurements were found to be in the target range of 5–10 mmol/l, also haemoglobin levels were higher with the IV infusion regimen, although chest X-rays revealed no infective processes either pre- or postoperatively.[302] Alternatively the insulin to glucose ratio was significantly lower in people receiving IV insulin compared to the subcutaneous group, and the number of dosage adjustments required was lower with the IV delivery method.[303] No significant hyper- or hypoglycaemic events were recorded in either trial (**Ib**).

The use of a two pump IV infusion technique in which a y-shaped cannula was connected to separate pumps delivering glucose and potassium and another providing insulin was compared to a standard IV regimen with variable amounts of insulin being added to a glucose and potassium infusion bag during a range of surgical procedures on people with Type 1 diabetes.[304] The former method provided lower glucose concentrations when people were being taken off infusion during the sliding scale period, and when on their normal insulin regimen postoperatively as compared to the standard method. However there were no significant differences between groups in the median length of time on the regimens, the length of stay or in the number of infections reported (**Ib**).

An experimental method for adjusting dose of infused insulin for critically ill diabetic patients using a fuzzy logic principle compared with standard algorithms was tested in a small randomised controlled trial.[305] Over 72 hours the adjustment using fuzzy logic produced lower mean blood glucose levels than the standard method, with level falling below 10 mmol/l in a shorter period. This appeared to be achieved by more frequent dose adjustments (**Ia**).

Myocardial infarction

A large randomised controlled trial including 620 people[306] demonstrated a significant reduction in total mortality at three months, one year and three and a half years, and re-infarctions following insulin-glucose infusion, compared to controls (**Ib**).

One moderate-sized prospective randomised trial in an elderly mixed diabetic population (19% Type 1)[307] tested the use of 24 hours of infused insulin, followed by subcutaneous injections for three months. This was found to reduce glucose levels further than a control of no insulin during the first 24 hours of admission. However no significant differences in HbA_{1c} were noted between the group to 24 hours. There was also excess incidence of hypoglycaemia among the insulin-treated patients (**Ia**).

An additional prospective controlled trial[308] showed a significant reduction in total mortality and the occurrence of complications (heart failure and arrhythmias) with continuous intravenous insulin therapy compared to conventional therapy, however, this population was predominantly people with Type 2 diabetes. Subgroup analysis showed that reductions in complications were only significant in patients treated with oral hypoglycaemic agents, no insulin or diet alone (**IIa**).

▷ Health economic evidence

One UK-based study[297] suggested that the provision of a hospital-based diabetes specialist nurse lowered the cost per patient admission without producing a significant difference in readmission, quality of life or patient satisfaction.

▷ Consideration

The evidence supporting the benefit of specialist multidisciplinary team advice in giving healthcare and cost gains to inpatients outside specialist diabetes wards was felt to be conclusive. Professional and patient members of the group were sadly familiar with the failure of some wards to use the expertise of people with diabetes, and the distress this can cause when care becomes suboptimal as a result. This was noted to be particularly the case in relation to nutritional intake and insulin therapy.

The evidence base for optimal use of insulin therapy in people with diabetes suffering critical acute arterial (and non-arterial) emergencies comes mainly from cohorts of people with Type 2 diabetes. The pathophysiological situation in these circumstances was not thought to be significantly different in Type 1 diabetes, and that evidence was therefore taken as the basis for a clinical recommendation.

The group was aware that the most widely established technique for managing people requiring insulin through surgical and other procedures (the glucose–insulin–potassium infusion) was not identified by the literature search despite a significant descriptive literature. Nevertheless, the prevalent use of this technique throughout the UK was felt to be such that it would be inappropriate not to recommend its general use.

RECOMMENDATIONS

R160   From the time of admission, the person with Type 1 diabetes and the team caring for   B
        him or her should receive, on a continuing basis, advice from a trained
        multidisciplinary team with expertise in diabetes.

R161   Throughout the course of an inpatient admission, the personal expertise of adults   D
        with Type 1 diabetes (in managing their own diabetes) should be respected and
        routinely integrated into ward-based blood glucose monitoring and insulin delivery,
        using the person with Type 1 diabetes' own system. This should be incorporated into the
        nursing care plan.

R162   Throughout the course of an inpatient admission, the personal knowledge and needs   D
        of adults with Type 1 diabetes regarding their dietary requirements should be a major
        determinant of the food choices offered to them (except when illness or medical or
        surgical intervention significantly disturbs those requirements).

R163   Hospitals should ensure the existence and deployment of an approved protocol for   D
        inpatient procedures and surgical operations for adults with Type 1 diabetes. This
        should aim to ensure the maintenance of near-normoglycaemia without risk of acute
        decompensation, usually by the use of regular quality-assured blood glucose testing
        driving the adjustment of intravenous insulin delivery.

R164   Members of care teams managing adults with Type 1 diabetes in institutions, such as   D
        nursing homes, residential homes and prisons, should follow the recommendations
        in this section.

Management during acute arterial events

R165   Optimal insulin therapy, which can be achieved by the use of intravenous insulin and   D
        glucose, should be provided to all adults with Type 1 diabetes with threatened or actual
        myocardial infarction or stroke. Critical care and emergency departments should have a
        protocol for such management.

13.4   Associated illness

▷   Rationale

Type 1 diabetes is an auto-immune disease associated with genes which modulate the immune response. Other auto-immune diseases are similarly associated, and manifestation of some of them can be sub-clinical while interacting with aspects of food absorption or metabolism.

▷   Evidence statements

Latent pernicious anaemia

Using a microbiological method to measure cobalamin concentration, one study from Australia[309] found reduced cobalamin concentration in six out of 371 people with Type 1 diabetes. Four of the patients showed no clinical signs of pernicious anaemia, the fifth was mildly anaemic and the sixth patient was not available for further testing. This medium-sized study with methodological limitations gave a prevalence of latent pernicious anaemia of 11 per 1000 in people with Type 1 diabetes (**III**).

Prevalence of coeliac disease

Using immunoglobulin A (IgA) class anti-endomysial antibodies (EmAb) detected by immunofluorescence (test) and histological confirmation of coeliac disease by small intestinal biopsy partial or total villous atrophy, a medium-sized study[310] showed in an unselected sample at an outpatients clinic that the prevalence of coeliac disease in the sampled population was 6.4% and that EmA were highly predictive of the presence of coeliac disease on biopsy (**DS**).

A larger study,[311] but with potential methodological limitations, found that in a two-step screening process of anti-gliadin antibodies (GA) detected by enzyme-linked immunosorbent assay (ELISA) assay and IgA class EmAb detected by immunofluorescence, the predictive value of GA was moderate, with a high false-positive rate for IgA-GA. Prevalence of coeliac disease in Type 1 diabetes to be up to 2.6% and that after 30 years diabetes duration, the prevalence of coeliac disease was >6%. The study also found that EmAb were highly predictive of the presence of coeliac disease on biopsy (**DS**).

The frequency of coeliac disease-specific serologic markers and the prevalence of coeliac disease in families of patients with Type 1 diabetes were evaluated in a medium-sized study[312] using a two-step screening process. The screening programme included circulating islet cell antibodies (ICA), anti-glutamic acid decarboxylase antibodies and GA, and then IgA class EmAb detected by immunofluorescence. This study found the prevalence of biopsy-proven coeliac disease to be 1.3% among patients with Type 1 diabetes and zero among controls, or family. Of screening assays, only EmAb were highly predictive of the presence of coeliac disease (**DS**).

Another diagnostic study using IgA class EmAb[313] compared people with Type 1 diabetes with adults with coeliac disease as true positives (as determined by intestinal biopsy) and controls (healthy and diseased) as true negatives (as determined by intestinal biopsy). The prevalence of biopsy-proven coeliac disease among adults with Type 1 diabetes was 3.13%. This study showed IgA class EmAb had high specificity in detecting coeliac disease in people with Type 1 diabetes (**DS**).

Red cell distribution width

Using red cell distribution width (RDW) as a screening test against EmAb and diagnostic duodenal biopsy as reference tests for coeliac disease one very small, methodologically-limited study[314] demonstrated the poor specificity of RDW in predicting coeliac disease in people with Type 1 diabetes. Given the potential methodological limitations, this evidence was not used to support any recommendations in this area (**DS**).

▷ Health economic evidence

The health economic searches found no relevant papers for the treatment of those with Type 1 diabetes suffering from concurrent disease.

▷ Consideration

While auto-immune conditions are probably more common in people with Type 1 diabetes than in the general population, the group did not feel that this should lead to any formal system of surveillance for the development of such conditions.

RECOMMENDATIONS

R166   In adults with Type 1 diabetes of low body mass index or with unexplained weight loss,   **DS**
markers of coeliac disease should be assessed.

R167   Healthcare professionals should be alert to the possibility of development of other   **D**
auto-immune disease in adults with Type 1 diabetes (including Addison's disease,
pernicious anaemia and thyroid disorders).

13.5   Psychological problems

▷ Rationale

The management demands of insulin therapy, the risks of late complications of diabetes, and the problems of hypoglycaemia and social discrimination, can place significant emotional stress on people with Type 1 diabetes. This might precipitate or exacerbate psychological difficulties present for other reasons. Additionally, the stresses might in themselves be expected to interfere with a person's ability to self-manage their diabetes.

▷ Evidence statements

Depressed mood and glycaemic control

A small cohort study examining depressed mood as a factor in glycaemic control in Type 1 diabetes[315] found a strong positive correlation between mood and glycaemic control. As the depression scores for this sample were mainly in the normal range, the results of this study indicate that mood, rather than clinical depression *per se*, is associated with significant differences in glycaemic control (**IIa**).

A medium-sized cohort study[316] examined depression and its effect on reporting diabetes symptoms in Type 1 diabetes. The study found that seven of nine symptoms attributed to diabetes (hyperglycaemic symptoms, hypoglycaemic symptoms and non-specific symptoms of poor control) were associated with depression whereas only one of nine symptoms attributed to diabetes was related to HbA_1 (**IIa**).

A meta-analysis of cross-sectional studies[317] examined whether depression is associated with glycaemic control. A weak correlation was found between depression and glycaemic control. However, the study has certain potential issues with the methodology used. No systematic quality appraisal has been given for those studies included in the meta-analysis. Effect size estimates may be unstable due to the small number of studies and the small sample sizes of some studies (**III**).

Injection anxiety and glycaemic control

One medium-sized cohort study[318] examined 'fear of blood and injury' and its association with glycaemic control in Type 1 diabetes. The study shows that Type I diabetes adults with poorer glycaemic control perform fewer blood glucose measurements per day. The relationship between poor glycaemic control and fewer blood glucose measurements is mediated by fear of blood and injury (**IIa**).

Another medium-sized cohort study[319] examined injection anxiety in Type 1 and Type 2 diabetes. The study found a significant negative correlation between injection anxiety and the number of insulin injections. However, no significant difference was found in the degree of glycaemic control between diabetes patients with high *vs* low anxiety scores. The results of this study are not analysed separately for people with Type 1 and Type 2 diabetes (**III**).

One meta-analysis[320] examined whether or not anxiety is associated with poor glycaemic control in adults with Type 1 and Type 2 diabetes. The studies that were limited to Type 1 diabetes found a weak correlation between anxiety and glycaemic control. However, the study has some possible methodological limitations which may have introduced bias into analysis. No systematic quality appraisal has been given for those studies included in the meta-analysis. Effect size estimates may be unstable due to the small number of studies and the small sample sizes of some studies (**III**).

Prevalence of depression in Type I diabetes

One recent meta-analysis of prevalence studies examining the prevalence of depression in Type 1 diabetes[321] found a significantly higher prevalence of depression in Type 1 diabetes (21.7%) than in non-diabetes control subjects (8.6%). Potential methodological factors inherent to the study may limit the validity of the results derived from the meta-analysis (**III**).

One retrospective cross-sectional case-control study[322] examined the prevalence of antidepressant use in Type 1 diabetes compared to age- and sex-matched controls. The study found a significantly higher proportion of Type 1 diabetes patients (12.8%) had received a prescription for antidepressants in the past twelve months compared to controls (7.4%). The data for this study was derived from a localised computerised database of 28 GP practices so caution needs to be taken when generalising these results to other geographical areas (**III**).

Management of depression

A medium-sized prospective 12-month follow-up study in Type 1 diabetes[323] evaluated whether a blood glucose awareness training programme (BGAT-2) would improve mood. No significant improvement in mood was detected in baseline scores at six and 12 months. This is attributed to baseline scores being within the normal limits. When subjects who feel within the range of mild depression were examined separately, these individuals did demonstrate a significant reduction in baseline scores at six and 12 months (**IIb**).

A small randomised controlled trial[324] evaluated the efficacy of nortriptyline for depression and poor glycaemic control in a mixed (Type 1 and Type 2) diabetes population with poor glycaemic control. The study found that the nortriptyline group were significantly less depressed after eight weeks than the placebo-treated patients. Of the nortriptyline-treated patients, 57% successfully remitted compared to 35.7% of the placebo-treated patients. No significant difference in response rate was found between Type 1 and Type 2 diabetes. Furthermore, in the sample as a whole (Type 1 and Type 2) there was a non-significant trend towards worsened glycaemic control, both in patients who received nortriptyline and those who received placebo (**Ib**).

A small randomised controlled trial[325] evaluated the antidepressant efficacy of fluoxetine in diabetic patients (mixed population type sample) with major depressive disorder. At the conclusion of the eight-week treatment period, a significant reduction in symptoms of depression was found in the fluoxetine-treated group compared to the placebo group. However, no significant difference in the improvement of glycaemic control was found between patients who received fluoxetine and those who received placebo (**Ib**).

A small random two-group parallel comparison with a pre-test and nine and 15 months follow-up study[326] compared the effects of a standard intensive treatment, patient education and distress reduction programme, with a standard treatment and patient education. Outcomes examined were psychological variables and metabolic control. At nine months follow-up, depression improved significantly in the intensive treatment group compared to the standard treatment group. No significant difference was found in metabolic control between the two groups. At 15 months follow-up, improvement in depression faded and metabolic control was worsened (**Ib**).

Management of anxiety in Type 1 diabetes

A small double-blind randomised controlled trial in a mixed (Type 1 and Type 2) diabetes population[327] examined the effects of alprazolam on glucose regulation in anxious and non-anxious patients with poor glycaemic control. Patients treated with alprazolam had a significantly greater reduction in GHb levels than those receiving placebo, regardless of anxiety. Both alprazolam and placebo similarly improved anxiety among anxious patients. Results were not analysed separately for Type 1 and Type 2 diabetes (**Ib**).

▷ Consideration

It was felt that, whether or not depression and other psychological illness was more common in people with Type 1 diabetes, the literature being inconclusive, the interaction with self-management demanded professional alertness to such problems. A degree of competence in managing these problems at least matching that of an experienced general practitioner is clearly desirable.

RECOMMENDATIONS

R168   Members of professional teams providing care or advice to adults with Type 1 diabetes   **B**
should be alert to the development or presence of clinical or sub-clinical depression and/or anxiety, in particular where someone reports or appears to be having difficulties with self-management.

R169   Diabetes professionals should ensure they have appropriate skills in the detection and   **D**
basic management of non-severe psychological disorders in people from different cultural backgrounds. They should be familiar with appropriate counselling techniques and appropriate drug therapy, while arranging prompt referral to specialists of those people in whom psychological difficulties continue to interfere significantly with well-being or diabetes self-management.

R170   Special management techniques or treatment for non-severe psychological illness   **D**
should not commonly be used, except where diabetes-related arterial complications give rise to special precautions over drug therapy.

13.6   Eating disorders

▷   Rationale

Due to the inadequacies of subcutaneous insulin therapy, dietary self-management is an inevitable consequence of the optimal self-care of Type 1 diabetes. Eating disorders are not uncommon in the general population, while Type 1 diabetes is most commonly diagnosed at an age (12–20) when consciousness of own body image is high. Accordingly, eating disorders are seen in people with Type 1 diabetes, and will interfere with self-management.

A review of the management of eating disorders is outside the scope of this guideline. A systematic search of the literature was, however, undertaken to review the types and relevant prevalence of eating disorders, and whether any specific issues of management had been identified in the Type 1 diabetes population.

▷   Evidence statements

Many papers on eating disorders in diabetes include people with Type 2 diabetes. Extrapolation to Type 1 diabetes from such populations is not safe. Assessment of eating disorders can be by interview (specific, low prevalence) or questionnaire (non-specific, high prevalence), and may or may not include manipulation of insulin dosage (dose omission or reduction). Accordingly published prevalence and odds ratio *vs* matched populations vary. Furthermore there may be cultural variations depending on attitudes to obesity and peer pressure. People with diabetes often are in continued contact with professional care teams, and the input of those teams might be expected to have influence on behavioural disorders (**IV**).

A follow-up study using interview methods in a clinic population[328] found no eating disorders at all. Nevertheless a proportion of young people did use insulin dose manipulation to control weight, and appeared to have worse outcomes (markers of late complications of diabetes) as a result (III).

A group in Toronto published a series of papers over the last decade, including a non-systematic review.[329–30] They note the odds ratio for eating disorders in young people compared to non-diabetic controls is around 2.0, with an excess prevalence of 2%–5%. The principal disorders described are bulimia nervosa and insulin dose manipulation, the conditions tend to be chronic even under care, and diabetes outcomes relatively poor compared to peers (III).

A review,[331] described as a meta-analysis of prevalence studies, concurred with these figures for bulimia and dose manipulation, and could not find evidence of increased prevalence of anorexia nervosa (III).

One small randomised controlled trial of a group psycho-education programme to improve sub-clinical disordered eating in women with Type 1 diabetes[332] found no significant differences between the intervention and control (standard care) in outcomes of metabolic control with both groups showing improvements from baseline. There was also no significant difference in concordance with diabetes treatment or eating disorder symptomology at six weeks (Ib).

A position statement of the American Dietetic Association and the Dietitians of Canada[333] found evidence that the prevalence of eating disorders among young adult women with Type 1 diabetes to be about 5% to 11%. It is suggested that dietetic professionals have a vital role in the management of diabetes as they have an understanding of the health issues that affect women with diabetes (IV).

▷ Consideration

The group felt that the evidence on the whole suggested that eating disorders were more prevalent in people with Type 1 diabetes, and particularly in young adults. Insulin dose manipulation of calorie loss accounted for much of this, and perhaps the long-term follow-up study's results were influenced by the benefits of the good long-term support offered. Experience of eating disorders in clinical practice was that in the context of insulin therapy they can have serious short- and long-term impacts, sometimes fatal.

RECOMMENDATIONS

R171   Members of multidisciplinary professional teams should be alert to the possibility of   C
        bulimia nervosa, anorexia nervosa and insulin dose manipulation in adults with Type 1
        diabetes with:
        ● over-concern with body shape and weight
        ● low body mass index
        ● poor overall blood glucose control.

R172   The risk of morbidity from the complications of poor metabolic control suggests that   D
        consideration should be given to early (and occasionally urgent) referral of adults with
        Type 1 diabetes to local eating disorder services.

R173   Provision for high-quality professional team support at regular intervals with regard to   D
counselling about lifestyle issues and particularly nutritional behaviour should be
made for all adults with Type 1 diabetes from the time of diagnosis (see section 6.1,
'Education programmes for adults with Type 1 diabetes' and 6.3, 'Dietary management').

14 | Areas for future research

Priority areas

- ❑ Comparative studies of education models from the time of diagnosis of Type 1 diabetes.
- ❑ Use of well-being and treatment satisfaction assessment tools to enhance the patient-professional interface and make care more directed to the agenda of adults with Type 1 diabetes, while improving biomedical outcomes.
- ❑ A study of multiple interventions to reduce arterial and microvascular risk in adults with Type 1 diabetes identified as being at high risk of development or progression of the late complications.
- ❑ Long-term assessment of recall systems allowing longer intervals between complication/risk factor detection visits according to assessed risk.
- ❑ Trials of regimens and duration of traditional antibiotic therapies in adults with neuropathic foot ulceration.
- ❑ Studies of the effectiveness of quality assurance systems in the surveillance of late complications.

Other areas

- ❑ Cognitive behavioural therapy for adults with very poor glucose control without obvious organic cause.
- ❑ Development of assessment interviews and questionnaires designed for eating disorders in adults with Type 1 diabetes.
- ❑ Epidemiological studies of trends in the incidence of late complications in defined populations of adults with Type 1 diabetes.
- ❑ Role of lipid-lowering drugs in the prevention of arterial disease in adults with Type 1 diabetes, and studies of markers of higher risk.
- ❑ Models of care for the primary prevention of foot ulceration in adults with Type 1 diabetes.
- ❑ Studies of the economics of the combined and fragmented annual review system.
- ❑ Studies of skill substitution for the initial assessment of diabetes eye photographs in diabetes eye screening.
- ❑ Studies of different methods of day-to-day and meal-to-meal adjustment of insulin doses using defined insulin regimens and appropriate educational packages.
- ❑ Trials of combined renin-angiotensin system blockers in progressive diabetic nephropathy
- ❑ Studies of the optimal use of the new rapid-acting and extended-acting insulins.
- ❑ Approaches to the management of hypoglycaemia unawareness using the new insulins.
- ❑ Assessment of the economic burden of Type 1 diabetes in defined populations.
- ❑ Assessment of the reliability and patient acceptability of self-monitoring of blood glucose in the context of specific regimens.
- ❑ Comparative studies of alternate site and traditional site self-glucose monitoring including patient satisfaction measures.

❑ Studies of the role of continuous glucose monitoring systems.

❑ Means of surveillance for, and treatment of, sexual dysfunction in women with Type 1 diabetes.

❑ Trials of different insulin regimens for people with poor glycaemic control despite apparently optimal education and self-care.

❑ Robust studies of the efficacy of the oral glucose-lowering agents, metformin and insulin sensitisers.

❑ Development of a useful arterial risk equation specifically for adults with Type 1 diabetes.

APPENDICES

Appendix A: Clinical questions and search strategies

Reference made to the Cochrane Library in the table below is inclusive of the following; Cochrane Systematic Reviews database, CENTRAL and DARE. The Cochrane Systematic Reviews database contains items that are constantly updated. CENTRAL contains items resulting from searches performed in the process of creating Cochrane Sytemtematic Reviews and goes back as far as the Cochrane searches to date. The DARE database was set up by the NHS Centre for Reviews and Dissemination in 1994. It does, however, include records that have an earlier publication date. For example, it contains a set of records from a systematic reviews database maintained by the UK Cochrane Centre prior to 1995. This set of records is no longer updated and has not been assessed by the NHS's Centre for Reviews and Dissemination.

Table A1 Clinical questions and search strategies

Question	Population	Study type	Database and year
1 Introduction			
Q1 What is the working clinical definition for Type 1 diabetes?			Expert review
Q2 What is the current burden and trend in burden of Type 1 diabetes in England and Wales?			Expert review
4 Diagnosis			
Q3 What symptoms are suggestive of a diagnosis of Type 1 diabetes?			Expert review
Q4 Which diagnostic tests can confirm diagnosis in a person with suspected Type 1 diabetes?			Expert review
5 Care structure and delivery			
Q5 What is the evidence on optimal structures of care, which enable healthcare professionals to give assistance, education and advice to adults with Type 1 diabetes?	Adults T1DM	All studies	Cochrane Library 1980–2003 Medline 1980–2003 Embase 1980–2003 CINAHL 1982–2003
Q6 What support groups help adults with Type 1 diabetes and their families to cope with diabetes?			Expert review
6 Patient education and self-care			
Q7 What are the optimal methods of delivering education to adults with Type 1 diabetes?	Adults T1DM	Systematic reviews	Cochrane Library 1980–2003
		RCTs, cohorts	Medline 1980–2003 Embase 1980–2003 CINAHL 1982–2003 PsychINFO 1980–2003

continued

Table A1 Clinical questions and search strategies – *continued*

Question	Population	Study type	Database and year
6 Patient education and self-care – *continued*			
Q8 In adults with Type 1 diabetes, what are the optimal methods to improve concordance with self-management?	Adults T1DM	Systematic reviews	Cochrane Library 1980–2003
		RCTs, cohorts	Medline 1980–2003 Embase 1980–2003 CINAHL 1982–2003 PsychINFO 1980–2003
Q9 What is the optimum form of self-monitoring of glucose control in adults with Type 1 diabetes? Q10 What is the optimum regimen of self-monitoring of glucose control in adults with stable Type 1 diabetes?	Adults T1DM	Systematic reviews	Cochrane Library 1977–2003
		RCTs, cohorts	Medline 1977–2003 Embase 1980–2003 CINAHL 1982–2003
Q11 What dietary advice should be given to adults with Type 1 diabetes to maintain optimal metabolic control?	Adults T1DM	Systematic reviews	Cochrane Library 1980–2003
		RCTs, cohorts	Medline 1980–2003 Embase 1980–2003 CINAHL 1982–2003
Q12 & Q13 Questions removed.			
Q14 What advice about exercise participation should be given to adults with Type 1 diabetes to maintain optimal blood glucose control?	Adults T1DM	Systematic reviews	Cochrane Library 1985–2003
		RCTs, cohorts	Medline 1985–2003 Embase 1985–2003 CINAHL 1985-2003
Q15 Question removed.			
Q20 What recommendations can be made for the special needs of members of minority ethnic communities with diabetes?		Expert review	
Q21 What precautions and lifestyle changes do adults living with Type 1 diabetes need to make to maintain metabolic control?		Expert review	
7 Blood glucose control and insulin therapy			
Q22 What is an acceptable level of blood glucose control in adults with Type 1 diabetes for the avoidance of complications?		Expert review	
Q23 What are the optimal methods of managing glucose control in inpatients with stable Type 1 diabetes?	Adults T1DM	Systematic reviews	Cochrane Library 1980–2003
		RCTs, cohorts	Medline 1980–2003 Embase 1980–2003 CINAHL 1982–2003
Q25 What is the optimum method of clinically monitoring blood glucose control? Q26 What is the optimum frequency of clinically monitoring blood glucose control?	Adults T1DM	Systematic reviews	Cochrane Library 1977–2003
		RCTs, cohorts	Medline 1977–2003 Embase 1980–2003 CINAHL 1982–2003
Q68 In newly-diagnosed adults with Type 1 diabetes (excluding those still requiring hospital inpatient treatment) what initial insulin regimens aid glycaemic control?	Adults T1DM	Systematic reviews	Cochrane Library 1980–2003
		RCTs	Medline 1980–2003 Embase 1980–2003 CINAHL 1982–2003

continued

Table A1 Clinical questions and search strategies – *continued*

Question	Population	Study type	Database and year
7 Blood glucose control and insulin therapy – *continued*			
Q27 What types of insulin regimen aid optimal diabetic control in adults with stable Type 1 diabetes?			
Q29 In adults with Type 1 diabetes and poorly-controlled blood glucose what insulin regimens can improve diabetic control?			
Q28 What specific advice can be given to adults with Type 1 diabetes for the management and prevention of hypoglycaemia?	Adults T1DM	Systematic reviews	Cochrane Library 1980–2003
		RCTs, cohorts	Medline 1980–2003 Embase 1980–2003 CINAHL 1982-2003
Q30 What method of insulin delivery aids optimal diabetic control in adults with stable Type 1 diabetes? Q31 In adults with Type 1 diabetes and poorly-controlled blood glucose what methods of insulin delivery can improve diabetic control?	Adults T1DM	Systematic reviews	Cochrane Library 1980–2003
		RCTs	Medline 1980–2003 Embase 1980–2003 CINAHL 1982–2003
Q32 Are there sub-groups of adults with Type 1 diabetes who need a different insulin delivery method to aid optimal diabetic control?			Expert review
Q33 Can combination therapy (oral glucose lowering drugs and insulin) improve blood glucose control compared to insulin therapy alone in adults with Type 1 diabetes?	Adults T1DM	Systematic reviews	Cochrane Library 1980–2003
		RCTs	Medline 1980–2003 Embase 1980–2003
Q34 Question removed.			
Q71 What is the most appropriate medical intervention for adults with Type 1 diabetes with severe hypoglycaemia?	Adults T1DM	Systematic reviews	Cochrane Library
		RCTs, cohorts	Medline 1966–2003 Embase 1980–2003
8 Arterial risk control			
Q35 What is an acceptable level of blood pressure control in adults with Type 1 diabetes?			Expert review
Q36 In adults with Type 1 diabetes and hypertension, what is optimum intervention to lower blood pressure?	Adults T1DM	Systematic reviews	Cochrane Library 1980–2003
		RCTs	Medline 1980–2003 Embase 1980–2003
Q37 What is the optimum method of surveillance for arterial risk factors in adults with Type 1 diabetes? Q38 What are the screening tests for arterial risk factors in adults with Type 1 diabetes?	Adults T1DM, non-diabetes systematic reviews	Systematic reviews	Cochrane Library 1990–2003
		RCTs, cohorts	Medline 1990–2003 Embase 1990–2003
Q39 What is an acceptable level of lipid control in adults with Type 1 diabetes?			Expert review
Q40 In adults with Type 1 diabetes, what is the optimum method for predicting cardiovascular disease risk?	Adults T1DM	All study types	Cochrane Library 1990–2003 Medline 1990–2003 Embase 1990–2003

continued

Table A1 Clinical questions and search strategies – *continued*

Question	Population	Study type	Database and year
8 Arterial risk control – *continued*			
Q41 What is the optimum method of management of abnormalities in lipid control in adults with Type 1 diabetes?	Adults T1DM	Systematic reviews	Cochrane Library 1990–2003
		RCTs	Medline 1990–2003 Embase 1990-2003
Q42 What is the evidence for the use of antiplatelet agents in the prevention of arterial disease in adults with Type 1 diabetes?	Adults T1DM	Systematic reviews	Cochrane Library 1990–2003
		RCTs	Medline 1990–2003 Embase 1990–2003
Q43 In adults with Type 1 diabetes, what is the management of cardiovascular disease?	Adults T1DM	Systematic reviews	Cochrane Library 1990–2003
		RCTs	Medline 1990–2003 Embase 1990–2003
9 Management of complications: diabetic eye disease			
Q44 What is the optimum method for surveillance for diabetic eye damage in adults with Type 1 diabetes? Q45 What screening tests should be used for diabetic eye damage in adults with Type 1 diabetes?	Adults T1DM	Systematic reviews	Cochrane Library 1985–2003
		RCTs, cohorts	Medline 1985–2003 Embase 1985–2003 CINAHL 1985–2003
Q46 What non-laser, non-surgical means can be used to prevent the development of diabetic eye disease? Q47 What non-laser, non-surgical means can be used to slow the progression of diabetic eye disease?	Adults T1DM	Systematic reviews	Cochrane Library 1985–2003
		RCTs	Medline 1985–2003 Embase 1985–2003
Q48 When should an adult with Type 1 diabetes and diabetic eye damage be referred to an ophthalmologist?	Adults T1DM	Systematic reviews	Cochrane Library
		RCTs, cohorts	Medline 1966–2003 Embase 1980–2003 CINAHL 1982–2003
10 Management of complications: diabetic kidney disease			
Q49 In adults with Type 1 diabetes what is the optimum method of surveillance for the detection of emerging diabetic kidney disease? Q50 In adults with Type 1 diabetes what are the screening tests for emerging diabetic kidney disease?	Adults T1DM	Systematic reviews	Cochrane Library 1980–2003
		RCTs, cohorts	Medline 1980–2003 Embase 1980–2003 CINAHL 1982–2003
Q51 What is the appropriate management of early diabetic kidney disease in adults with Type 1 diabetes?	Adults T1DM	Systematic reviews	Cochrane Library 1980–2003
		RCTs	Medline 1980–2003 Embase 1980–2003
Q52 When should adults with early symptoms of diabetic kidney disease be referred to a renal specialist?	Adults T1DM	Systematic reviews	Cochrane Library 1980–2003
		RCTs, cohorts	Medline 1980–2003 Embase 1980–2003 CINAHL 1982–2003

continued

Table A1 Clinical questions and search strategies – *continued*

Question	Population	Study type	Database and year
11 Management of complications: diabetes foot problems			
Q53 In adults with Type 1 diabetes, what are the optimum methods for surveillance for diabetic foot problems?	Adults T1DM	Systematic reviews	Cochrane Library
		RCTs, cohorts	Medline 1966–2003 Embase 1980–2003 CINAHL 1982–2003
Q54 In adults with Type 1 diabetes, what are the optimum screening tests for diabetic foot problems?			
Q55 What are the optimum methods of managing diabetic foot problems in adults with Type 1 diabetes?	Adults T1DM	Systematic reviews	Cochrane Library
		RCTs	Medline 1966–2003 Embase 1980–2003 CINAHL 1982–2003 (no results before 1994)
Q56 In adults with Type 1 diabetes, what is the optimum treatment of foot ulceration and related infection?			
12 Management of complications: diabetes nerve damage			
Q57 In adults with Type 1 diabetes, what is the optimum management of painful neuropathy?	Adults T1DM	Systematic reviews	Cochrane Library 1980–2003
		RCTs	Medline 1980–2003 Embase 1980–2003
Q58 In adults with Type 1 diabetes, what are the symptoms suggestive of a diagnosis of autonomic neuropathy?	Adults T1DM	Systematic reviews	Cochrane Library 1980–2003
		RCTs, cohorts	Medline 1980–2003 Embase 1980–2003
Q59 What is the optimum method of managing autonomic neuropathy in adults with Type 1 diabetes?	Adults T1DM	Systematic reviews	Cochrane Library 1980–2003
		RCTs	Medline 1980–2003 Embase 1980–2003
Q60 In adults with Type 1 diabetes, what are the symptoms suggestive of a diagnosis of gastroparesis?	Adults T1DM	Systematic reviews	Cochrane Library 1980–2003
		RCTs, cohorts	Medline 1980–2003 Embase 1980-2003
Q61 What is the optimum method for surveillance for sexual dysfunction in adults with Type 1 diabetes?	Adults T1DM	Systematic reviews	Cochrane Library 1980–2003
		RCTs	Medline 1966–2003 Embase 1980–2003
Q62 What are the optimum methods of management for sexual dysfunction in adults with Type 1 diabetes?			
Q63 & 64 Questions removed.			
13 Management of special situations			
Q16 How are adults with Type 1 diabetes affected by anxiety and depression?	Adults T1DM	Systematic reviews	Cochrane Library 1980–2003
		RCTs, cohorts	Medline 1980–2003 Embase 1980–2003 CINAHL 1982–2003 PsychINFO 1980–2003
Q17 How best is such anxiety and depression diagnosed and managed in adults with Type 1 diabetes?			
Q18 What is the best means of detecting eating disorders in adults with Type 1 diabetes?			Expert review

continued

Table A1 Clinical questions and search strategies – *continued*

Question	Population	Study type	Database and year
13 Management of special situations – *continued*			
Q19 What is the appropriate management of eating disorders in adults with Type 1 diabetes?	Adults T1DM	Systematic reviews	Cochrane Library 1980–2003
		RCTs, cohorts	Medline 1980–2003 Embase 1980–2003 CINAHL 1982–2003 PsychINFO 1980–2003
Q24 What is the optimum management of blood glucose and metabolic control in adults with Type 1 diabetes suffering myocardial infarction and cardiovascular accident?	Adults T1DM	Systematic reviews	Cochrane Library 1980–2003
		RCTs, cohorts	Medline 1980–2003 Embase 1980–2003 CINAHL 1982–2003
Q65 What is the recommended initial assessment plan for newly-diagnosed adults with stable Type 1 diabetes?	Adults T1DM	Guidelines	WWW 1985
Q66 What is the recommended initial content of education to promote understanding of Type 1 diabetes and improve self-management in newly-diagnosed adults with stable Type 1 diabetes? Q67 What is the recommended delivery of education to promote understanding of Type 1 diabetes and improve initial self-management of newly-diagnosed adults with stable Type 1 diabetes?	Adults T1DM	Systematic reviews	Cochrane Library 1980–2003
		RCTs, cohorts	Medline 1980–2003 Embase 1980–2003 CINAHL 1982–2003
Q69 Question removed.			
Q70 What guidance can be given for optimal insulin delivery during severe concurrent illness?	Adults T1DM	Systematic reviews	Cochrane Library 1980–2003
		RCTs, cohorts	Medline 1980–2003 Embase 1980–2003 CINAHL 1982–2003
Q72 In people with diabetic ketoacidosis what emergency care can reduce morbidity and mortality?	Adults T1DM	Systematic reviews	Cochrane Library 1970–2003
		RCTs, cohorts	Medline 1970–2003 Embase 1980–2003 CINAHL 1982–2003
Q73 What is the most appropriate surveillance and screening for concurrent autoimmune diseases in adults with Type 1 diabetes?	Adults T1DM	All studies	Cochrane Library Medline 1966–2003 Embase 1980–2003 CINAHL 1982–2003
Q74 What are the optimal insulin regimes during surgical procedures?	Adults T1DM	Systematic reviews	Cochrane Library 1980–2003
		RCTs	Medline 1980–2003 Embase 1980–2003

Appendix B: Unlicensed medicines

The following medicines in this guideline are not licensed for the management of Type 1 diabetes (or its common complications, signs or symptoms) in the UK at the time of issue:

- **aspirin** is licensed for primary and secondary prevention of arterial disease, but not specifically for arterial risk associated with Type 1 diabetes
- **carbamazepine** is licensed for trigeminal neuralgia but not for painful neuropathy associated with Type 1 diabetes
- **cisapride** is not licensed in the UK and any prescription will have to be made in consultation with the pharmacist
- **intravenous insulin and/or glucose/potassium** is licensed for 'urgent treatment', not explicitly for Type 1 diabetes management following stroke or myocardial infarction
- **phenytoin** is licensed for neuropathic pain under specialist supervision
- **phosphate** replacement is not licensed for diabetic ketoacidosis
- **tricyclic and related antidepressants** (amitriptyline, amoxapine, clomipramine, dosulepin (dothiepin), doxepin, imipramine, lofepramine, maprotiline, mianserin, nortriptyline, trazodone and trimipramine) are not licensed for painful neuropathy associated with Type 1 diabetes.

Appendix C: The scope of the guideline

Guideline title

Type 1 diabetes: diagnosis and management of type 1 diabetes in primary and secondary care*

Short title

Type 1 diabetes

Background

- ❑ The National Institute for Clinical Excellence ('NICE' or 'the Institute') has commissioned the National Collaborating Centre for Women and Children's Health to develop a clinical guideline on type 1 diabetes for babies, children and adolescents, and the National Collaborating Centre for Chronic Conditions to develop a clinical guideline on type 1 diabetes for adults and older people for use in the NHS in England and Wales. This follows referral of the topic by the Department of Health and Welsh Assembly Government (see below). The guideline will provide recommendations for good practice that are based on the best available evidence of clinical and cost-effectiveness.
- ❑ The Institute's clinical guidelines will support the implementation of national service frameworks (NSFs) in those aspects of care where a framework has been published. The statements in each NSF reflect the evidence that was used at the time the framework was prepared. The clinical guidelines and technology appraisals published by the Institute after an NSF has been issued will have the effect of updating the framework.

Clinical need for the guideline

- ❑ Type 1 diabetes is a continuing hormonal deficiency disorder that has significant impact on lifestyle in the short term, and is associated with major long-term complications and reduced life expectancy. People with type 1 diabetes require insulin replacement therapy.
- ❑ Diabetes is estimated to affect 2% of the general population. There are over 1 million people with diagnosed diabetes in England and Wales (and perhaps a similar number with undiagnosed diabetes). Type 1 diabetes accounts for about 15%–20% of cases.
- ❑ Good blood glucose and blood pressure control are known to prevent or delay the long-term complications of diabetes.
- ❑ Systems of surveillance for the early detection of complications are important as is effective management of late complications when they occur.

---

*This title, and the short title, were subsequently changed while the guideline was being prepared for publication.

The guideline

- ❑ The guideline development process is described in detail in three booklets that are available from the NICE website (see 'Further information'). *The guideline development process: information for stakeholders* describes how organisations can become involved in the development of a guideline.
- ❑ This document is the scope. It defines exactly what this guideline will (and will not) examine, and what the guideline developers will consider. The scope is based on the referral from the Department of Health and Welsh Assembly Government (see below).
- ❑ The guideline will take into account the results of the related technology appraisals being carried out by the Institute, which include insulin pump therapy (due for publication April 2003) and patient education models for diabetes (due for publication March 2003).
- ❑ The areas that will be addressed by the guideline are described in the following sections.

Population

▷ Groups that will be covered

- ❑ The guideline will address the diagnosis and management of babies, children, adolescents, adults and older people with type 1 diabetes.

▷ Groups that will not be covered

- ❑ The guideline will not address the specific management of women with diabetes who wish to conceive or who are pregnant.
- ❑ The guideline will not address the management of women who develop diabetes during pregnancy because consideration will be given to developing a separate guideline on diabetes in pregnancy (covering type 1 diabetes, type 2 diabetes and gestational diabetes).

▷ Healthcare setting

- ❑ The guideline will cover the care received from primary and secondary healthcare professionals who have direct contact with and make decisions concerning the care of people with type 1 diabetes.
- ❑ The guideline will address the interface between community and specialist care including the circumstances in which people should be referred or admitted to specialist care.
- ❑ The guideline will pay particular attention to the interface between paediatric and adult services.
- ❑ The guideline will address the support/advice that the NHS should offer to crèches, nurseries, schools and other institutions.
- ❑ The guideline will also be relevant to the work but will not cover the practice of:
  - social services and the voluntary sector
  - services supplied by secondary and tertiary specialties for late complications of diabetes (for example, renal, cardiology, urology, ophthalmology services) to whom patients have been referred
  - the education sector (eg schools and universities).

Clinical management

The guideline will cover the following aspects of management.

❑ Diagnosis, including detection before deterioration to an emergency state, assessment of the degree of acute severity, and assurance of the type of diabetes. Screening for high-risk groups will not be included.

❑ Diagnostic and monitoring techniques, including:
- glycated haemoglobin
- self-monitoring
- testing for ketones
- lipids
- blood pressure
- systems of continuous glucose monitoring.

❑ Pharmacological treatments, including:
- the different types and species of natural and synthetic insulins, and their combination in different insulin regimens
- means of insulin delivery, taking into account the needs of special groups
- acarbose.

Advice on treatment options will be based on the best evidence available to the development group. When referring to pharmacological treatments, the guideline will normally make recommendations within the licensed indications. Exceptionally, and only where the evidence supports it, the guideline may recommend use outside the licensed indications. The guideline will assume that prescribers will use the Summary of Product Characteristics to inform their prescribing decisions for individual patients.

❑ Non-pharmacological management, including:
- dietary interventions and management
- patient education techniques (taking account of the Institute's technology appraisal)
- carer education techniques
- special needs of adolescents
- other lifestyle management including physical activity, smoking cessation and diet.

❑ Psychosocial factors with consideration to the support needed by patients, parents and carers:
- at the time of diagnosis with type 1 diabetes
- in relation to maximising people's ability to achieve good glycaemic control
- for the prevention of complications, via improved control
- in relation to adjustment to complications that occur
- in relation to the identification and treatment of psychiatric disorders (particularly depressive disorders) that are known to have an impact on control and, therefore, outcome
- in people identified as having particularly severe difficulties with living with their diabetes, whether in primary or secondary healthcare settings.

❑ Management of special situations, including the management of:
- hypoglycaemia and hypoglycaemic coma
- diabetic ketoacidosis
- intercurrent illnesses including the avoidance of severe hyperglycaemia

- those people on non-diabetes hospital wards
- those undergoing procedures including peri-operative care
- those in institutional care.

❑ The guideline will address surveillance for developing complications, interventions to prevent complications and the early and ongoing management of complications for the following conditions taking into account the Institute's guideline on type 2 diabetes. These will include:

- active surveillance of children with diabetes for associated conditions, especially coeliac disease and hypothyroidism
- retinopathy
- foot risk factors including peripheral vascular disease and neuropathy
- developing nephropathy
- cardiovascular risk factors and ischaemic heart disease
- impotence and erectile dysfunction
- dental problems
- neuropathies.

❑ Methods to optimise blood glucose control and blood pressure control and quality of life.

❑ Guidance to ensure that patients and carers have the information they need and the opportunities to discuss with their clinicians the advantages and disadvantages of treatment so that they can make informed choices about their treatment. This will include specific information about diabetes and the role of self-help groups where evidence exists.

Audit support within guideline

The guideline will incorporate review criteria and audit advice.

The audit should complement other existing and proposed work of relevance, including the Diabetes Information Strategy to be linked to the Diabetes National Service Framework, the National Clinical Audit Database and the Institute's guidelines on type 2 diabetes.

Status

▷ Scope

This is the final version of the scope.

▷ Guideline

The development of the guideline recommendations will begin in Spring 2002.

Further information

Information on the guideline development process is provided in:

- *The guideline development process: information for the public and the NHS*
- *The guideline development process: information for stakeholders*
- *The guideline development process: information for National Collaborating Centres and Guideline Development Groups*

These booklets are available as PDF files from the NICE website (**www.nice.org.uk**). Information on the progress of the guideline will also be available from the website.

Referral from the Department of Health and Welsh Assembly Government

The Department of Health and Welsh Assembly Government asked the Institute to address the following topics in the guideline:

- initial management at diagnosis including admission criteria and initial insulin regimes
- ongoing monitoring of glycaemic control, including the role of home glucose monitoring and the frequency of HbA_{1c} measurement
- prevention and management of ketoacidosis, including the management of intercurrent illness
- management of hypoglycaemia and hypoglycaemic coma
- peri-operative management of patients with type 1 diabetes
- management of type 1 diabetes during pregnancy
- surveillance for complications.

As with other topics, we would like this guideline to have an associated audit methodology which will help to change practice and improve care for patients:

- the number of people with type 1 diabetes who have experienced one (or more) episodes of ketoacidosis in the last year
- the proportion of people with type 1 diabetes whose HbA_{1c} levels have been stabilised at less that 7% one year after diagnosis.

Appendix D: Evidence tables

These are available at **www.rcplondon.ac.uk/pubs/books/dia/index.asp**

The evidence tables provide full details of the studies identified and critically appraised as part of the formal systematic review. They are organised according to guideline section, clinical question and study design.

References

1. Gray A, Fenn P, McGuire A. The cost of insulin-dependent diabetes mellitus (IDDM) in England and Wales. *Diabetic Medicine* 1995;**12**:1068–76.

2. Currie C, Peters J. Costs of insulin-dependent diabetes mellitus. *Diabetic Medicine* 1996;**13**:684–5.

3. Evans JM, MacDonald TM, Leese GP *et al.* Impact of type 1 and type 2 diabetes on patterns and costs of drug prescribing: a population-based study. *Diabetes Care* 2000;**23**:770–4.

4. National Institute for Clinical Excellence. *Information for National Collaborating Centres and Guideline Development Groups.* The Guideline Development Process Series No. 3. London: NICE, 2004.

5. Home PD, Coles J, Goldacre M *et al.* *Health outcome indicators: Diabetes. A report of a working group to the Department of Health.* Oxford: National Centre for Health Outcomes Development, 1999.

6. Eccles M, Mason J. How to develop cost-conscious guidelines. *Health Technology Assessment* 2001;**5**:1–69.

7. Murphy MK, Black NA, Lamping DL *et al.* *Consensus development methods and their use in clinical guideline development,* 1998.

8. World Health Organization. *Definition, diagnosis, and classification of diabetes mellitus and its complications. Report of a WHO consultation. Part 1: Diagnosis and classification of diabetes mellitus.* Geneva: WHO, 1999.

9. Delahanty L, Simkins SW, Camelon K. Expanded role of the dietitian in the Diabetes Control and Complications Trial: implications for clinical practice. The DCCT Research Group. *Journal of the American Dietetic Association* 1993;**93**:758–64, 767.

10. Loveman E, Royle P, Waugh N. *Specialist nurses in diabetes mellitus.* The Cochrane Library, 2003.

11. Sadur CN, Moline N, Costa M *et al.* Diabetes management in a health maintenance organization. Efficacy of care management using cluster visits. *Diabetes Care* 1999;**22**:2011–7.

12. Thompson DM, Kozak SE, Sheps S. Insulin adjustment by a diabetes nurse educator improves glucose control in insulin-requiring diabetic patients: a randomized trial. *Canadian Medical Association Journal* 1999;**161**:959–62.

13. Hearnshaw H, Hopkins J, Wild A *et al.* Mandatory, multidisciplinary education in diabetes care. Can it meet the needs of primary care organisations? *Practical Diabetes International* 2001;**18**:274–80.

14. Koblik T, Sieradzki J, Friedlein J, Legutko J. First Polish multidisciplinary diabetic foot team: results of the first three years of operation – the Cracow study. *Diabetologia Polska* 1999;**6**:233–8.

15. Larsson J, Apelqvist J, Agardh CD, Stenstrom A. Decreasing incidence of major amputation in diabetic patients: a consequence of a multidisciplinary foot care team approach? *Diabetic Medicine* 1995;**12**:770–6.

16. Brink SJ, Miller M, Moltz KC. Education and multidisciplinary team care concepts for pediatric and adolescent diabetes mellitus. *Journal of Pediatric Endocrinology and Metabolism* 2002;**15**:1113–30.

17. Yokoyama KK, Cryar AK, Griffin KC *et al.* Cost-effectiveness of a multidisciplinary diabetes care clinic. *Drug Benefit Trends* 2002;**14**:36–44.

18. Dargis V, Pantelejeva O, Jonushaite A *et al.* Benefits of a multidisciplinary approach in the management of recurrent diabetic foot ulceration in Lithuania: a prospective study. *Diabetes Care* 1999;**22**:1428–31.

19. Cox D, Gonder-Frederick L, Polonsky W *et al.* A multicenter evaluation of blood glucose awareness training – II. *Diabetes Care* 1995;**18**:523–8.

20. Apelqvist J, Ragnarson-Tennvall G, Persson U, Larsson J. Diabetic foot ulcers in a multidisciplinary setting. An economic analysis of primary healing and healing with amputation. *Journal of Internal Medicine* 1994;**235**:463–71.

21. Frykberg RG. Team approach toward lower extremity amputation prevention in diabetes. *Journal of the American Podiatric Medical Association* 1997;**87**:305–12.

22. Riazi A, Hammersley S, Eiser C *et al.* Patients' experiences of the diabetes annual review. *Practical Diabetes International* 2000;**17**:226–30.

23. Braid E, Campbell B, Curtis S *et al.* The diabetes annual review as an educational tool: assessment and learning integrated with care, screening, and audit. *Diabetic Medicine* 1992;**9**:389–94.

24. International Diabetes Foundation. *A guide to type 1 (insulin dependent) diabetes mellitus.* Brussels: IDF, 1998.

25. Grabert M, Schweiggert F, Holl RW. A framework for diabetes documentation and quality management in Germany: 10 years of experience with DPV. *Computer Methods and Programs in Biomedicine* 2002;**69**: 115–21.

26. Azzopardi J, Fenech FF, Junoussov Z *et al.* A computerized health screening and follow-up system in diabetes mellitus. *Diabetic Medicine* 1995;**12**:271–6.

27. Burnett SD, Woolf CM, Yudkin JS. Developing a district diabetic register. *British Medical Journal* 1992; **305**:627–30.

28. Burnett SD, Press M, Yudkin JS. Compiling a district diabetic register: theoretical and practical considerations. *Diabetic Medicine* 1993;**10**:199–200.

29. Elwyn GJ, Vaughan NJ, Stott NC. District diabetes registers: more trouble than they're worth? Review. *Diabetic Medicine* 1998;**15**(Suppl 3):S44–8.

30. Harris MF, Priddin D, Ruscoe W *et al.* Quality of care provided by general practitioners using or not using division-based diabetes registers. *Medical Journal of Australia* 2002;**177**:250–2.

31. Howitt AJ, Cheales NA. Diabetes registers: a grassroots approach. *British Medical Journal* 1993;**307**:1046–8.

32. Kelly W, Bilous R, Murray G. A comprehensive register for diabetic outpatients: experience with desktop computing from 1987–1996. *Computer Methods and Programs in Biomedicine* 1998;**56**:205–10.

33. Coppell K, Manning P; Otago Diabetes Team. Establishing a regional diabetes register and a description of the registered population after one year. *New Zealand Medical Journal* 2002;**115**:U146.

34. Kleschen MZ, Holbrook J, Rothbaum AK *et al.* Improving the pneumococcal immunization rate for patients with diabetes in a managed care population: a simple intervention with a rapid effect. *Joint Commission Journal on Quality Improvement* 2000;**26**:538–46.

35. Kopelman PG, Michell JC, Sanderson AJ. DIAMOND: a computerized system for the management and evaluation of district-wide diabetes care. *Diabetic Medicine* 1995;**12**:83–7.

36. Vaughan NJ, Shaw M, Boer F *et al.* Creation of a District Diabetes Register using the DIALOG system. Review. *Diabetic Medicine* 1996;**13**:175–81.

37. Day JL, Metcalfe J, Johnson P. Benefits provided by an integrated education and clinical diabetes centre: a follow-up study. *Diabetic Medicine* 1992;**9**:855–9.

38. Bridgford A, Davis TM. A comprehensive patient-held record for diabetes. Part one: Initial development of the Diabetes Databank. *Practical Diabetes International* 2001;**18**:241–5.

39. Davis TM, Bridgford A. A comprehensive patient-held record for diabetes. Part two: Large-scale assessment of the diabetes databank by patients and health care workers. *Practical Diabetes International* 2001;**18**:311–4.

40. Engelbrecht R, Hildebrand C, Kuhnel E *et al.* A chip card for patients with diabetes. *Computer Methods and Programs in Biomedicine* 1994;**45**:33–5.

41. Engelbrecht R, Hildebrand C, Brugues E *et al.* DIABCARD – an application of a portable medical record for persons with diabetes. *Medical Informatics* 1996;**21**:273–82.

42. Engelbrecht R, Hildebrand C. DIABCARD a smart card for patients with chronic diseases. *Clinical Performance and Quality Health Care* 1997;**5**:67–70.

43. Engelbrecht R, Hildebrand C. Telemedicine and diabetes. *Studies in Health Technology and Informatics* 1999;**64**:142–54.

44. Fischer U, Salzsieder E, Menzel R *et al.* Primary health care of diabetic patients in a specialized outpatient setting: a DIABCARE-based analysis. *Diabète et Métabolisme* 1993;**19**:188–94.

45. Chiarelli F, Verrotti A, Di Ricco L, LaPorte RE. Information superhighway, Internet and diabetes. *Diabetes, Nutrition and Metabolism – Clinical and Experimental* 1998;**11**:219–24.

46. Gorman C, Looker J, Fisk T *et al.* A clinically useful diabetes electronic medical record: lessons from the past; pointers toward the future. Review. *European Journal of Endocrinology* 1996;**134**:31–42.

47. Piwernetz K, Renner R, Mohrlein A *et al.* Analysis and processing of data in a hospital-based diabetes management system. *Hormone and Metabolic Research Supplement* 1990;**24**:109–15.

48. Smith SA, Murphy ME, Huschka TR *et al.* Impact of a diabetes electronic management system on the care of patients seen in a subspecialty diabetes clinic. *Diabetes Care* 1998;**21**:972–6.

49. Stroebel RJ, Scheitel SM, Fitz JS *et al.* A randomized trial of three diabetes registry implementation strategies in a community internal medicine practice. *Joint Commission Journal on Quality Improvement* 2002;**28**:441–50.

50. Biermann E, Dietrich W, Rihl J, Standl E. Are there time and cost savings by using telemanagement for patients on intensified insulin therapy? A randomised, controlled trial. *Computer Methods and Programs in Biomedicine* 2002;**69**:137–46.

51. McGill M, Constantino M, Yue DK. Integrating telemedicine into a National Diabetes Footcare Network. *Practical Diabetes International* 2000;**17**:235–8.

52. Cummings DM, Morrissey S, Barondes MJ *et al.* Screening for diabetic retinopathy in rural areas: the potential of telemedicine. *Journal of Rural Health* 2001;**17**:25–31.

53. McCulloch DK. Impact of endocrine and diabetes team consultation on hospital length of stay for patients with diabetes. *Diabetes Spectrum* 1996;**9**:180–1. [Commentary on Levetan CS, Salas R, Wiltes IF *et al. American Journal of Medicine* 1995;**99**:22–8].

54. Levetan CS, Salas JR, Wilets IF, Zumoff B. Impact of endocrine and diabetes team consultation on hospital length of stay for patients with diabetes. *American Journal of Medicine* 1995;**99**:22–8.

55. Koproski J, Pretto Z, Poretsky L. Effects of an intervention by a diabetes team in hospitalized patients with diabetes. *Diabetes Care* 1997;**20**:1553–5.

56. Hentinen M, Kyngas H. Diabetic adolescents' compliance with health regimens and associated factors. *International Journal of Nursing Studies* 1996;**33**:325–37.

57. Kaplan RM, Hartwell SL. Differential effects of social support and social network on physiological and social outcomes in men and women with type II diabetes. *Health Psychology* 1987;**6**:387–98.

58. Fisher L, Chesla CA, Bartz RJ *et al.* The family and type 2 diabetes: a framework for intervention. *Diabetes Educator* 1998;**24**:599–607.

59. Hanson CL, Henggeler SW, Burghen GA. Social competence and parental support as mediators of the link between stress and metabolic control in adolescents with insulin-dependent diabetes mellitus. *Journal of Consulting and Clinical Psychology* 1987;**55**:529–33.

60. Schafer LC, McCaul KD, Glasgow RE. Supportive and nonsupportive family behaviors: relationships to adherence and metabolic control in persons with type I diabetes. *Diabetes Care* 1986;**9**:179–85.

61. Bailey BJ, Kahn A. Apportioning illness management authority: how diabetic individuals evaluate and respond to spousal help. *Qualitative Health Research* 1993;**3**:55–73.

62. The DAWN (Diabetes Attitudes, Wishes and Needs) Study. *Practical Diabetes International* 2002;**19**:22a–4a.

63. Diabetes UK and Care Interventions Team. *Needs of the recently diagnosed. Listening project. Report and recommendations.* London: Diabetes UK, 2001.

64. Hiscock J, Legard R, Snape D. *Listening to Diabetes Service Users: Qualitative findings for the Diabetes National Service Framework.* London: Department of Health, 2003.

65. Assessing the benefit of support groups. *New England Journal of Medicine* 2001;**345**:1719–68.

66. Knight BG, Lutzky SM, Macofsky-Urban F. A meta-analytic review of interventions for caregiver distress: recommendations for future research. *Gerontologist* 1993;**33**:240–8.

67. Toseland RW, Labrecque MS, Gobel ST, Whitney MH. An evaluation of a group program for spouses of frail elderly veterans. *Gerontologist* 1992;**32**:382–90.

67a. Data obtained from an email from Debbie Hammond, Diabetes UK patients representative on the Guideline Development Group, August 2003.

68. Labrecque MS, Peak T. Long-term effectiveness of a group program for caregivers of frail elderly veterans. *American Journal of Orthopsychiatry* 1992;**62**:575–88.

69. Ostwald SK, Hepburn KW, Caron W *et al.* Reducing caregiver burden: a randomized psychoeducational intervention for caregivers of persons with dementia. *Gerontologist* 1999;**39**:299–309.

70. Hanestad BR, Albrektsen G. The effects of participation in a support group on self assessed quality of life in people with insulin-dependent diabetes mellitus. *Diabetes Research and Clinical Practice* 1993;**19**:163–73.

71. Maxwell AE, Hunt IF, Bush MA. Effects of a social support group, as an adjunct to diabetes training, on metabolic control and psychosocial outcomes. *Diabetes Educator* 1992;**18**:303–9.

72. Fisher EB, Auslander WF, Munro JF *et al.* Neighbors for a smoke free north side: Evaluation of a community organization approach to promoting smoking cessation among African Americans. *American Journal of Public Health* 1998;**88**:1658–63.

73. Morris DB. A rural diabetes support group. *Diabetes Educator* 1998;**24**:493–7.

74. Nuffield Trust. Sharing, stories: a feasibility study of facilitated small group learning by the oral tradition in diabetes education for British Bangladeshis in Tower Hamlets. 2000.

75. Home P, Coles J, Goldacre M *et al* (eds). *Health outcome indicators: diabetes mellitus.* Report of a working group to the Department of Health. Oxford: National Centre for Health outcomes Development, 1999.

76. American Diabetes Association. Standards of medical care for patients with diabetes mellitus. *Diabetes Care* 2003;**26**(Suppl 1):S33–50.

77. Carpentier WS, Piziak VK, Bratcher T, Hejl J. Efficacy of diabetes education: classroom versus individualized instruction. *HMO Practice* 1990;**4**:30–3.

78. Kim JY, Phillips TL. The effectiveness of two forms of corrective feedback in diabetes education. *Journal of Computer-Based Instruction* 1991;**18**:14–8.

79. Mensing C, Boucher J, Cypress M. National standards for diabetes self-management education. *Diabetes Care* 2003;**26**(Suppl 1):S149–56.

80. Rapid Reviews Team, Southampton Health Technology Assessment Centre, University of Southampton. *Patient education models for diabetes.* London: National Institute for Clinical Excellence, 2002.

81. de Weerdt I, Visser AP, Kok GJ *et al.* Randomized controlled multicentre evaluation of an education programme for insulin-treated diabetic patients: effects on metabolic control, quality of life, and costs of therapy. *Diabetic Medicine* 1991;**8**:338–45.

82. Lennon GM, Taylor KG, Debney L, Bailey CJ. Knowledge, attitudes, technical competence, and blood glucose control of Type 1 diabetic patients during and after an education programme. *Diabetic Medicine* 1990;**7**:825–32.

83. Valk GD, Kriegsman DM, Assendelft WJ. Patient education for preventing diabetic foot ulceration: a systematic review. *Endocrinology and Metabolism Clinics of North America* 2002;**31**:633–58.

84. Norris SL, Nichols PJ, Caspersen CJ *et al.* Increasing diabetes self-management education in community settings. A systematic review. *American Journal of Preventive Medicine* 2002;**22**:39–66.

85. Jones PM. Use of a course on self-control behavior techniques to increase adherence to prescribed frequency for self-monitoring blood glucose. *Diabetes Educator* 1990;**16**:296–303.

86. Matam P, Kumaraiah V, Munichoodappa C *et al.* Behavioural intervention in the management of compliance in young type-I diabetics. *Journal of the Association of Physicians of India* 2000;**48**:967–71.

87. Korhonen T, Huttunen JK, Aro A *et al.* A controlled trial on the effects of patient education in the treatment of insulin-dependent diabetes. *Diabetes Care* 1983;**6**:256–61.

88. Halimi S, Charpentier G, Grimaldi A *et al.* Effect on compliance, acceptability of blood glucose self-monitoring and HbA(1c) of a self-monitoring system developed according to patient's wishes. The ACCORD study. *Diabetes and Metabolism* 2001;**27**:681–7.

89. Coster S, Gulliford MC, Seed PT *et al.* Monitoring blood glucose control in diabetes mellitus: a systematic review. *Health Technology Assessment* 2000;**4**:No.12.

90. Germer S, Campbell IW. Home-monitoring of blood glucose – patient preference for 'BM-Test Glycemie 20–800' strips or 'Glucometer'. *British Journal of Clinical Practice* 1985;**39**:225–7.

91. Edelman SV, Callahan P, Deeb LC. Multisite evaluation of a new diabetes self-test for glucose and glycated protein (fructosamine) [including commentary by Riddle MC]. *Diabetes Technology and Therapeutics* 2000;**2**:233–40.

92. Cefalu WT, Wang ZQ, Redmon E *et al.* Clinical validity of a self-test fructosamine in outpatient diabetic management [including commentary by Hom F]. *Diabetes Technology and Therapeutics* 1999;**1**:435–45.

93. Gordon D, Semple CG, Paterson KR. Do different frequencies of self-monitoring of blood glucose influence control in type 1 diabetic patients? *Diabetic Medicine* 1991;**8**:679–82.

94. Giacco R, Parillo M, Rivellese AA *et al.* Long-term dietary treatment with increased amounts of fiber-rich low-glycemic index natural foods improves blood glucose control and reduces the number of hypoglycemic events in type 1 diabetic patients. *Diabetes Care* 2000;**23**:1461–6.

95. Hansen HP, Christensen PK, Tauber LE *et al.* Low-protein diet and kidney function in insulin-dependent diabetic patients with diabetic nephropathy. *Kidney International* 1999;**55**:621–8.

96. Chantelau EA, Frenzen A, Gosseringer G *et al.* Intensive insulin therapy justifies simplification of the diabetes diet: a prospective study in insulin-dependent diabetic patients. *American Journal of Clinical Nutrition* 1987;**45**:958–62.

97. McCulloch DK, Mitchell RD, Ambler J, Tattersall RB. A prospective comparison of 'conventional' and high carbohydrate/high fibre/low fat diets in adults with established type 1 (insulin-dependent) diabetes. *Diabetologia* 1985;**28**:208–12.

98. Yale JF, Begg I, Gerstein H *et al.* 2001 Canadian Diabetes Association clinical practice guidelines for the prevention and management of hypoglycemia in diabetes. *Canadian Journal of Diabetes Care* 2001;**26**:22–35.

99. Amiel S, Beveridge S, Bradley C *et al.* Training in flexible, intensive insulin management to enable dietary freedom in people with type 1 diabetes: dose adjustment for normal eating (DAFNE) randomised controlled trial. *British Medical Journal* 2002;**325**:746–9.

100. Muhlhauser I, Bott U, Overmann H *et al.* Liberalized diet in patients with type 1 diabetes. *Journal of Internal Medicine* 1995;**237**:591–7.

101. National Institute for Clinical Excellence. *Guidance on the use of patient-education models for diabetes.* London: NICE, 2003.

102. Laaksonen DE, Atalay M, Niskanen LK *et al.* Aerobic exercise and the lipid profile in type 1 diabetic men: a randomized controlled trial. *Medicine and Science in Sports and Exercise* 2000;**32**:1541–8.

103. Ligtenberg PC, Blans M, Hoekstra JB *et al.* No effect of long-term physical activity on the glycemic control in type 1 diabetes patients: a cross-sectional study. *Netherlands Journal of Medicine* 1999;**55**:59–63.

104. Lehmann R, Kaplan V, Bingisser R *et al.* Impact of physical activity on cardiovascular risk factors in IDDM. *Diabetes Care* 1997;**20**:1603–11.

105. Perry TL, Mann JI, Lewis-Barned NJ *et al.* Lifestyle intervention in people with insulin-dependent diabetes mellitus (IDDM). *European Journal of Clinical Nutrition* 1997;**51**:757–63.

106. Schneider SH, Khachadurian AK, Amorosa LF *et al.* Ten-year experience with an exercise-based outpatient life-style modification program in the treatment of diabetes mellitus. *Diabetes Care* 1992;**15**:1800–10.

107. Connor H, Annan F, Bunn E *et al.* The implementation of nutritional advice for people with diabetes. *Diabetic Medicine* 2003;**20**:786–807.

108. Larsen ML. The clinical usefulness of glucated haemoglobin in diabetes care evaluated by use of a medical technology assessment strategy. Review. *Danish Medical Bulletin* 1997;**44**:303–15.

109. Gross TM, Bode BW, Einhorn D *et al.* Performance evaluation of the MiniMed continuous glucose monitoring system during patient home use. *Diabetes Technology and Therapeutics* 2000;**2**:49–56.

110. Gross TM, Ter Veer A. Continuous glucose monitoring in previously unstudied population subgroups. *Diabetes Technology and Therapeutics* 2000;**2**(Suppl 1):S27–34.

111. Maran A, Crepaldi C, Tiengo A *et al.* Continuous subcutaneous glucose monitoring in diabetic patients: a multicenter analysis. *Diabetes Care* 2002;**25**:347–52.

112. Grieve R, Beech R, Vincent J, Mazurkiewicz J. Near patient testing in diabetes clinics: appraising the costs and outcomes. *Health Technology Assessment* 1999;**3**:1–74.

113. Wang PH, Lau J, Chalmers TC, Zinman B. Intensive blood-glucose control and diabetes: a meta-analysis. *Annals of Internal Medicine* 1993;**119**:71.

114. Alberti KG, Gries FA. Management of non-insulin-dependent diabetes mellitus in Europe: a consensus view. *Diabetic Medicine* 1988;**5**:275–81.

115. European Diabetes Policy Group. A desktop guide to Type 1 (insulin-dependent) diabetes mellitus. 1998. *Diabetic Medicine* 1999;**16**:253–66.

116. Rohlfing CL, Wiedmeyer HM, Little RR *et al.* Defining the relationship between plasma glucose and HbA(1c): analysis of glucose profiles and HbA(1c) in the Diabetes Control and Complications Trial. *Diabetes Care* 2002;**25**:275–8.

117. The effect of intensive treatment of diabetes on the development and progression of long-term complications in insulin-dependent diabetes mellitus. The Diabetes Control and Complications Trial Research Group. *New England Journal of Medicine* 1993;**329**:977–86.

118. The relationship of glycemic exposure (HbA1c) to the risk of development and progression of retinopathy in the diabetes control and complications trial. *Diabetes* 1995;**44**:968–83.

119. Stratton IM, Kohner EM, Aldington SJ *et al.* UKPDS 50: risk factors for incidence and progression of retinopathy in Type II diabetes over 6 years from diagnosis. *Diabetologia* 2001;**44**:156–63.

120. McCance DR, Hadden DR, Atkinson AB *et al.* Long-term glycaemic control and diabetic retinopathy. *Lancet* 1989;**ii**:824–8.

121. Reichard P, Nilsson BY, Rosenqvist U. The effect of long-term intensified insulin treatment on the development of microvascular complications of diabetes mellitus. *New England Journal of Medicine* 1993;**329**:304–9.

122. Krolewski AS, Laffel LM, Krolewski M *et al.* Glycosylated hemoglobin and the risk of microalbuminuria in patients with insulin-dependent diabetes mellitus. *New England Journal of Medicine* 1995;**332**:1251–5.

123. Peters AL, Davidson MB, Schriger DL, Hasselblad V. A clinical approach for the diagnosis of diabetes mellitus: an analysis using glycosylated hemoglobin levels. Meta-analysis Research Group on the Diagnosis of Diabetes Using Glycated Hemoglobin Levels. *Journal of the American Medical Association* 1996;**276**: 1246–52.

124. McCance DR, Hanson RL, Charles MA *et al.* Comparison of tests for glycated haemoglobin and fasting and two hour plasma glucose concentrations as diagnostic methods for diabetes. *British Medical Journal* 1994;**308**:1323–8.

125. Nathan DM, Singer DE, Hurxthal K, Goodson JD. The clinical information value of the glycosylated hemoglobin assay. *New England Journal of Medicine* 1984;**310**:341–6.

126. Richter B, Neises G, Bergerhoff K. Human versus animal insulin in people with diabetes mellitus: a systematic review. *Endocrinology and Metabolism Clinics of North America* 2002;**31**:723–49.

127. George E, Bedford C, Peacey SR *et al.* Further evidence for a high incidence of nocturnal hypoglycaemia in IDDM: no effect of dose for dose transfer between human and porcine insulins. *Diabetic Medicine* 1997;**14**:442–8.

128. Karlson B, Agardh CD. Influence of intensified insulin regimen on quality of life and metabolic control in insulin-dependent diabetes mellitus. *Diabetes Research and Clinical Practice* 1994;**25**:111–5.

129. Egger M, Davey G, Stettler SC, Diem P. Risk of adverse effects of intensified treatment in insulin-dependent diabetes mellitus: a meta-analysis. *Diabetic Medicine* 1997;**14**:919–28.

130. Haakens K, Hanssen KF, Dahl-Jorgensen K *et al.* Early morning glycaemia and the metabolic consequences of delaying breakfast/morning insulin. A comparison of continuous subcutaneous insulin infusion and multiple injection therapy with human isophane or human ultralente insulin at bedtime in insulin-dependent diabetics. *Scandinavian Journal of Clinical and Laboratory Investigation* 1989;**49**:653–9.

131. Tunbridge FK, Newens A, Home PD *et al.* Double-blind crossover trial of isophane (NPH)- and lente-based insulin regimens. *Diabetes Care* 1989;**12**:115–9.

132. National Institute for Clinical Excellence. *Guidance on the use of long-acting analogues for the treatment of diabetes – insulin glargine.* Technology Appraisal Guidance No.53. London: NICE, 2002.

133. Vignati L, Anderson JH Jr, Iversen PW. Efficacy of insulin lispro in combination with NPH human insulin twice per day in patients with insulin-dependent or non-insulin-dependent diabetes mellitus. Multicenter Insulin Lispro Study Group. *Clinical Therapeutics* 1997;**19**:1408–21.

134. Nielsen FS, Jorgensen LN, Ipsen M *et al.* Long-term comparison of human insulin analogue B10Asp and soluble human insulin in IDDM patients on a basal/bolus insulin regimen. *Diabetologia* 1995;**38**:592–8.

135. Lindholm A, McEwen J, Riis AP. Improved postprandial glycemic control with insulin aspart. A randomized double-blind cross-over trial in type 1 diabetes. *Diabetes Care* 1999;**22**:801–5.

136. Del Sindaco P, Ciofetta M, Lalli C *et al.* Use of the short-acting insulin analogue lispro in intensive treatment of type 1 diabetes mellitus: importance of appropriate replacement of basal insulin and time-interval injection-meal. *Diabetic Medicine* 1998;**15**:592–600.

137. Davey P, Grainger D, MacMillan J *et al.* Clinical outcomes with insulin lispro compared with human regular insulin: a meta-analysis. *Clinical Therapeutics* 1997;**19**:656–74.

138. Lalli C, Ciofetta M, Del Sindaco P *et al.* Long-term intensive treatment of type 1 diabetes with the short-acting insulin analog lispro in variable combination with NPH insulin at mealtime. *Diabetes Care* 1999;**22**:468–77.

139. Anderson JH Jr, Brunelle RL, Koivisto VA *et al.* Reduction of postprandial hyperglycemia and frequency of hypoglycemia in IDDM patients on insulin-analog treatment. Multicenter Insulin Lispro Study Group. *Diabetes* 1997;**46**:265–70.

140. Pfutzner A, Kustner E, Forst T *et al.* Intensive insulin therapy with insulin lispro in patients with type 1 diabetes reduces the frequency of hypoglycemic episodes. *Experimental and Clinical Endocrinology and Diabetes* 1996;**104**:25–30.

141. Renner R, Pfutzner A, Trautmann M *et al.* Use of insulin lispro in continuous subcutaneous insulin infusion treatment: results of a multicenter trial. *Diabetes Care* 1999;**22**:784–8.

142. Ebeling P, Jansson PA, Smith U *et al.* Strategies toward improved control during insulin lispro therapy in IDDM. Importance of basal insulin. *Diabetes Care* 1997;**20**:1287–9.

143. Roach P, Strack T, Arora V, Zhao Z. Improved glycaemic control with the use of self-prepared mixtures of insulin lispro and insulin lispro protamine suspension in patients with types 1 and 2 diabetes. *International Journal of Clinical Practice* 2001;**55**:177–82.

144. Gale EA. A randomized, controlled trial comparing insulin lispro with human soluble insulin in patients with Type 1 diabetes on intensified insulin therapy. The UK Trial Group. *Diabetic Medicine* 2000;**17**:209–14.

145. Roach P, Trautmann M, Arora V *et al.* Improved postprandial blood glucose control and reduced nocturnal hypoglycemia during treatment with two novel insulin lispro-protamine formulations, insulin lispro mix25 and insulin lispro mix50. Mix50 Study Group. *Clinical Therapeutics* 1999;**21**:523–34.

146. Holleman F, Schmitt H, Rottiers R *et al.* Reduced frequency of severe hypoglycemia and coma in well-controlled IDDM patients treated with insulin lispro. The Benelux-UK Insulin Lispro Study Group. *Diabetes Care* 1997;**20**:1827–32.

147. Ahmed AB, Home PD. The effect of the insulin analog lispro on nighttime blood glucose control in type 1 diabetic patients. *Diabetes Care* 1998;**21**:32–7.

148. Brunelle RL, Llewelyn J, Anderson JH *et al.* Meta-analysis of the effect of insulin lispro on severe hypoglycemia in patients with type 1 diabetes. *Diabetes Care* 1998;**21**:1726–31.

149. Shukla VK, Otten N. *Insulin lispro: a critical evaluation.* Ottawa: Canadian Coordinating Office for Health Technology Assessment; Issue 5, Feb 1999.

150. Home PD, Lindholm A, Hylleberg B, Round P. Improved glycemic control with insulin aspart: a multicenter randomized double-blind crossover trial in type 1 diabetic patients. UK Insulin Aspart Study Group. *Diabetes Care* 1998;**21**:1904–9.

151. Zinman B, Ross S, Campos RV, Strack T. Effectiveness of human ultralente versus NPH insulin in providing basal insulin replacement for an insulin lispro multiple daily injection regimen: a double-blind randomized prospective trial. *Diabetes Care* 1999;**22**:603–8.

152. Hermansen K, Madsbad S, Perrild H *et al.* Comparison of the soluble basal insulin analog insulin detemir with NPH insulin: a randomized open crossover trial in type 1 diabetic subjects on basal-bolus therapy. *Diabetes Care* 2001;**24**:296–301.

153. Stades AM, Hoekstra JB, van den Tweel I *et al*; STABILITY Study Group. Additional lunchtime basal insulin during insulin lispro intensive therapy in a randomized, multicenter, crossover study in adults: a real-life design. *Diabetes Care* 2002;**25**:712–7.

154. Fanelli CG, Pampanelli S, Porcellati F *et al.* Administration of neutral protamine Hagedorn insulin at bedtime versus with dinner in type 1 diabetes mellitus to avoid nocturnal hypoglycemia and improve control. A randomized, controlled trial. *Annals of Internal Medicine* 2002;**136**:504–14.

155. Dunbar JM, Madden PM, Gleeson DT *et al.* Premixed insulin preparations in pen syringes maintain glycemic control and are preferred by patients. *Diabetes Care* 1994;**17**:874–8.

156. DeVries JH, Snoek FJ, Kostense PJ *et al*; Dutch Insulin Pump Study Group. A randomized trial of continuous subcutaneous insulin infusion and intensive injection therapy in type 1 diabetes for patients with long-standing poor glycemic control. *Diabetes Care* 2002;**25**:2074–80.

157. Hollander P, Pi-Sunyer X, Coniff RF. Acarbose in the treatment of type I diabetes. *Diabetes Care* 1997;**20**:248–53.

158. Riccardi G, Giacco R, Parillo M *et al.* Efficacy and safety of acarbose in the treatment of Type 1 diabetes mellitus: a placebo-controlled, double-blind, multicentre study. *Diabetic Medicine* 1999;**16**:228–32.

159. Viviani GL, Camogliano L, Borgoglio MG *et al.* Acarbose treatment in insulin-dependent diabetics. A double-blind crossover study. *Current Therapeutic Research, Clinical Experimental* 1987;**42**:1–11.

160. Marena S, Tagliaferro V, Cavallero G *et al.* Double-blind crossover study of acarbose in type 1 diabetic patients. *Diabetic Medicine* 1991;**8**:674–8.

161. Gums JG, Curry RW Jr, Montes de Oca G *et al.* Treatment of type I diabetes with a combination of glyburide and insulin. *Annals of Pharmacotherapy* 1992;**26**:757–62.

162. Goldman J, Tamayo RC, Whitehouse FW, Kahkonen DM. Effect of glyburide on metabolic control and insulin binding in insulin-dependent diabetes mellitus. *Diabetes Care* 1984;**7**(Suppl 1):106–12.

163. Burke BJ, Hartog M, Waterfield MR. Improved diabetic control in insulin-dependent diabetics treated with insulin and glibenclamide. *Acta Endocrinologica* 1984;**107**:70–7.

164. Fallucca F, Sciullo E, Maldonato A. Combined therapy with insulin and sulfonylurea for the treatment of new-onset insulin-dependent diabetes mellitus. *Hormone and Metabolic Research* 1996;**28**:86–8.

165. National Institute for Clinical Excellence. *Guidance on the use of continuous subcutaneous insulin infusion for diabetes.* London: NICE, 2003.

166. Murray DP, Keenan P, Gayer E *et al.* A randomized trial of the efficacy and acceptability of a pen injector. *Diabetic Medicine* 1988;**5**:750–4.

167. Bantle JP, Neal L, Frankamp LM. Effects of the anatomical region used for insulin injections on glycemia in type I diabetes subjects. *Diabetes Care* 1993;**16**:1592–7.

168. de Meijer PH, Lutterman JA, van Lier HJ, van't Laar A. The variability of the absorption of subcutaneously injected insulin: effect of injection technique and relation with brittleness. *Diabetic Medicine* 1990;**7**: 499–505.

169. Fleming DR, Jacober SJ, Vandenberg MA *et al.* The safety of injecting insulin through clothing. *Diabetes Care* 1997;**20**:244–7.

170. Kinsley BT, Weinger K, Bajaj M *et al.* Blood glucose awareness training and epinephrine responses to hypoglycemia during intensive treatment in type 1 diabetes. *Diabetes Care* 1999;**22**:1022–8.

171. Fritsche A, Stumvoll M, Renn W, Schmulling RM. Diabetes teaching program improves glycemic control and preserves perception of hypoglycemia. *Diabetes Research and Clinical Practice* 1998;**40**:129–35.

172. Patrick AW, Collier A, Hepburn DA *et al.* Comparison of intramuscular glucagon and intravenous dextrose in the treatment of hypoglycaemic coma in an accident and emergency department. *Archives of Emergency Medicine* 1990;**7**:73–7.

173. Collier A, Steedman DJ, Patrick AW *et al.* Comparison of intravenous glucagon and dextrose in treatment of severe hypoglycemia in an accident and emergency department. *Diabetes Care* 1987;**10**:712–5.

174. Scottish Intercollegiate Guidelines Network. *Management of diabetes. A national clinical guideline.* SIGN Publication No.55. Edinburgh: SIGN, 2001.

175. Kanters SD, Banga JD, Stolk RP, Algra A. Incidence and determinants of mortality and cardiovascular events in diabetes mellitus: a meta-analysis. *Vascular Medicine* 1999;**4**:67–75.

176. Pignone MP, Phillips CJ, Atkins D *et al.* Screening and treating adults for lipid disorders. *American Journal of Preventive Medicine* 2001;**20**(3 Suppl):77–89.

177. Bayly GR, Bartlett WA, Davies PH *et al.* Laboratory-based calculation of coronary heart disease risk in a hospital diabetic clinic. *Diabetic Medicine* 1999;**16**:697–701.

178. Game FL, Bartlett WA, Bayly GR, Jones AF. Comparative accuracy of cardiovascular risk prediction methods in patients with diabetes mellitus. *Diabetes, Obesity and Metabolism* 2001;**3**:279–86.

179. Game FL, Jones AF. Coronary heart disease risk assessment in diabetes mellitus – a comparison of PROCAM and Framingham risk assessment functions. *Diabetic Medicine* 2001;**18**:355–9.

180. Jones AF, Walker J, Jewkes C *et al.* Comparative accuracy of cardiovascular risk prediction methods in primary care patients. *Heart* 2001;**85**:37–43.

181. Scottish Intercollegiate Guidelines Network. *Lipids and the primary prevention of coronary heart disease.* SIGN Publication No. 40. Edinburgh: SIGN, 1999.

182. Rustemeijer C, Schouten JA, Janssens EN *et al.* Pravastatin in diabetes associated hypercholesterolemia. *Acta Diabetologica* 1997;**34**:294–300.

183. Raskin P, Ganda OP, Schwartz S *et al.* Efficacy and safety of pravastatin in the treatment of patients with type I or type II diabetes mellitus and hypercholesterolemia. *American Journal of Medicine* 1995;**99**:362–9.

184. Goldberg RB, Mellies MJ, Sacks FM *et al.* Cardiovascular events and their reduction with pravastatin in diabetic and glucose-intolerant myocardial infarction survivors with average cholesterol levels: subgroup analyses in the cholesterol and recurrent events (CARE) trial. The Care Investigators. *Circulation* 1998;**98**:2513–9.

185. Sartor G, Katzman P, Eizyk E *et al.* Simvastatin treatment of hypercholesterolemia in patients with insulin dependent diabetes mellitus. *International Journal of Clinical Pharmacology and Therapeutics* 1995;**33**:3–6.

186. Hommel E, Andersen P, Gall MA *et al.* Plasma lipoproteins and renal function during simvastatin treatment in diabetic nephropathy. *Diabetologia* 1992;**35**:447–51.

187. Winocour PH, Durrington PN, Bhatnagar D *et al.* Double-blind placebo-controlled study of the effects of bezafibrate on blood lipids, lipoproteins, and fibrinogen in hyperlipidaemic type 1 diabetes mellitus. *Diabetic Medicine* 1990;**7**:736–43.

188. NHS Centre for Reviews and Dissemination. *Aspirin for the secondary prophylaxis of vascular disease in primary care.* Newcastle: University of Newcastle upon Tyne, Centre for Health Services Research; York: University of York, Centre for Health Economics, 1998.

189. ETDRS Investigators. Aspirin effects on mortality and morbidity in patients with diabetes mellitus. Early Treatment Diabetic Retinopathy Study report 14. *Journal of the American Medical Association* 1992;**268**: 1292–300.

190. Roffi M, Chew DP, Mukherjee D *et al.* Platelet glycoprotein IIb/IIIa inhibitors reduce mortality in diabetic patients with non-ST-segment-elevation acute coronary syndromes. *Circulation* 2001;**23**:2767–71.

191. Effects of ramipril on cardiovascular and microvascular outcomes in people with diabetes mellitus: results of the HOPE study and MICRO-HOPE substudy. Heart Outcomes Prevention Evaluation Study Investigators. *Lancet* 2000;**355**:253–9.

192. Yusuf S, Dagenais G, Pogue J *et al.* Vitamin E supplementation and cardiovascular events in high-risk patients. The Heart Outcomes Prevention Evaluation Study Investigators. *New England Journal of Medicine* 2000;**342**:154–60.

193. McAlister FA, Zarnke KB, Campbell NR *et al*; Canadian Hypertension Recommendations Working Group. The 2001 Canadian recommendations for the management of hypertension. Part two – therapy. *Canadian Journal of Cardiology* 2002;**18**:625–41.

194. Scottish Intercollegiate Guidelines Network. *Hypertension in older people.* SIGN Publication No. 49: Edinburgh: SIGN, 2001.

195. Adler AI, Stratton IM, Neil HA *et al.* Association of systolic blood pressure with macrovascular and microvascular complications of type 2 diabetes (UKPDS 36): prospective observational study. *British Medical Journal* 2000;**321**:412–9.

196. Ramsay L, Williams B, Johnston G *et al.* Guidelines for management of hypertension: report of the third working party of the British Hypertension Society. Review. *Journal of Human Hypertension* 1999;**13**: 569–92.

197. ALLHAT Officers and Coordinators for the ALLHAT Collaborative Research Group. The Antihypertensive and Lipid-Lowering Treatment to Prevent Heart Attack Trial. Major outcomes in high-risk hypertensive patients randomized to angiotensin-converting enzyme inhibitor or calcium channel blocker vs diuretic: The Antihypertensive and Lipid-Lowering Treatment to Prevent Heart Attack Trial (ALLHAT). *Journal of the American Medical Association* 2002;**288**:2981–97.

198. Schwartz SL, Hanson C, Lucas C *et al.* Double-blind, placebo-controlled study of ramipril in diabetics with mild to moderate hypertension. *Clinical Therapeutics* 1993;**15**:79–87.

199. Ferrier C, Ferrari P, Weidmann P *et al.* Swiss hypertension treatment programme with verapamil and/or enalapril in diabetic patients. *Drugs* 1992;**44**(Suppl 1):74–84.

200. Hutchinson A, McIntosh A, Peters J *et al.* Effectiveness of screening and monitoring tests for diabetic retinopathy – a systematic review. *Diabetic Medicine* 2000;**17**:495–506.

201. National Institute for Clinical Excellence. *Management of type 2 diabetes: retinopathy – screening and early management.* London: NICE, 2002:2.1.2.

202. Cummins E, Facey K, Macpherson K *et al.* *Health Technology Assessment of Organization of Services for Diabetic Retinopathy Screening (project).* Glasgow: Health Technology Board for Scotland, 2001.

203. Agence d'Evaluation des Technologies et des Modes d'Intervention en Santé. *Screening for diabetic retinopathy: validation of a system using telemedicine approach – primary research (project).* Quebec: AETMIS, 2002.

204. Pandit RJ, Taylor R. Quality assurance in screening for sight-threatening diabetic retinopathy. *Diabetic Medicine* 2002;**19**:285–91.

205. Mallamaci F, Zuccala A, Zoccali C *et al.* The deletion polymorphism of the angiotensin-converting enzyme is associated with nephroangiosclerosis. *American Journal of Hypertension* 2000;**13**:433–7.

206. Taylor R. Practical community screening for diabetic retinopathy using the mobile retinal camera: report of a 12 centre study. British Diabetic Association Mobile Retinal Screening Group. *Diabetic Medicine* 1996;**13**:946–52.

207. Frank RN. Aldose reductase inhibition. The chemical key to the control of diabetic retinopathy? *Archives of Ophthalmology* 1990;**108**:1229–31.

208. Ticlopidine treatment reduces the progression of nonproliferative diabetic retinopathy. The TIMAD Study Group. *Archives of Ophthalmology* 1990;**108**:1577–83.

209. Pagani A, Greco G, Tagliaferro V *et al.* Dipyridamole administration in insulin-dependent diabetics with background retinopathy: a 36-month follow-up. *Current Therapeutic Research, Clinical and Experimental* 1989;**45**:469–75.

210. Mota MC, Leite E, Ruas MA *et al.* Effect of cyclospasmol on early diabetic retinopathy. *International Ophthalmology* 1987;**10**:3–9.

211. Bursell SE, Clermont AC, Aiello LP *et al.* High-dose vitamin E supplementation normalizes retinal blood flow and creatinine clearance in patients with type 1 diabetes. *Diabetes Care* 1999;**22**:1245–51.

212. Tabaei BP, Al Kassab AS, Ilag LL *et al.* Does microalbuminuria predict diabetic nephropathy? *Diabetes Care* 2001;**24**:1560–6.

213. Almdal T, Norgaard K, Feldt-Rasmussen B, Deckert T. The predictive value of microalbuminuria in IDDM. A five-year follow-up study. *Diabetes Care* 1994;**17**:120–5.

214. Marshall SM, Collins A, Gregory W *et al.* Predictors of the development of microalbuminuria in patients with type I diabetes mellitus: a seven-year prospective study. *Diabetic Medicine* 1999;**16**:918–25.

215. Coonrod BA, Ellis D, Becker DJ *et al.* Predictors of microalbuminuria in individuals with IDDM. Pittsburgh Epidemiology of Diabetes Complications Study. *Diabetes Care* 1993;**16**:1376–83.

216. Yip JW, Jones SL, Wiseman MJ *et al.* Glomerular hyperfiltration in the prediction of nephropathy in IDDM: a 10-year follow-up study. *Diabetes* 1996;**45**:1729–33.

217. Mathiesen ER, Feldt-Rasmussen B, Hommel E *et al.* Stable glomerular filtration rate in normotensive IDDM patients with stable microalbuminuria. A 5-year prospective study. *Diabetes Care* 1997;**20**:286–9.

218. Ahn CW, Song YD, Kim JH *et al.* The validity of random urine specimen albumin measurement as a screening test for diabetic nephropathy. *Yonsei Medical Journal* 1999;**40**:40–5.

219. Ciavarella A, Silletti A, Forlani G *et al.* A screening test for microalbuminuria in type 1 (insulin-dependent) diabetes. *Diabetes Research and Clinical Practice* 1989;**7**:307–12.

220. Zelmanovitz T, Gross JL, Oliveira J, De Azevedo MJ. Proteinuria is still useful for the screening and diagnosis of overt diabetic nephropathy. *Diabetes Care* 2003;**21**:1076–9.

221. Ellis D, Coonrod BA, Dorman JS *et al.* Choice of urine sample predictive of microalbuminuria in patients with insulin-dependent diabetes mellitus. *American Journal of Kidney Diseases* 1989;**13**:321–8.

222. McHardy KC, Gann ME, Ross IS, Pearson DW. A simple approach to screening for microalbuminuria in a type 1 (insulin-dependent) diabetic population. *Annals of Clinical Biochemistry* 1991;**28**:450–5.

223. Collins AC, Vincent J, Newall RG *et al.* An aid to the early detection and management of diabetic nephropathy: assessment of a new point of care microalbuminuria system in the diabetic clinic. *Diabetic Medicine* 2001;**18**:928–32.

224. Shephard MD, Barratt LJ, Simpson-Lyttle W. Is the Bayer DCA 2000 acceptable as a screening instrument for the early detection of renal disease? *Annals of Clinical Biochemistry* 1999;**36**:393–4.

225. Webb DJ, Newman DJ, Chaturvedi N, Fuller JH. The use of the Micral-Test strip to identify the presence of microalbuminuria in people with insulin dependent diabetes mellitus (IDDM) participating in the EUCLID study. *Diabetes Research and Clinical Practice* 1996;**31**:93–102.

226. Agardh CD. A new semiquantitative rapid test for screening for microalbuminuria. *Practical Diabetes* 1993;**10**:146–7.

227. Adamson CL, Kumar S, Sutcliffe H *et al.* Screening strategies in the detection of microalbuminuria in insulin-dependent diabetic patients. *Practical Diabetes* 1993;**10**:142–4.

228. Gossain VV, Gunaga KP, Carella MJ *et al.* Utility of micral test strips in screening for microalbuminuria. *Archives of Pathology and Laboratory Medicine* 1996;**120**:1015–8.

229. Piehlmeier W, Renner R, Kimmerling T *et al.* Evaluation of the Micral-Test S, a qualitative immunologic patient self-test for microalbuminuria: the PROSIT project. Proteinuria Screening and Intervention. *Diabetic Medicine* 1998;**15**:883–5.

230. Kouri TT, Viikari JS, Mattila KS, Irjala KM. Microalbuminuria. Invalidity of simple concentration-based screening tests for early nephropathy due to urinary volumes of diabetic patients. *Diabetes Care* 1991;**14**:591–3.

231. Le Floch JP, Marre M, Rodier M, Passa P. Interest of Clinitek Microalbumin in screening for micro-albuminuria: results of a multicentre study in 302 diabetic patients. *Diabetes and Metabolism* 2001;**27**:36–9.

232. Lovell HG. *Angiotensin converting enzyme inhibitors in normotensive diabetic patients with microalbuminuria.* (Cochrane review). Cochrane Database of Systematic Reviews 2002; Issue 2, 2002.

233. ACE Inhibitors in Diabetic Nephropathy Trialist Group. Should all patients with type 1 diabetes mellitus and microalbuminuria receive angiotensin-converting enzyme inhibitors? A meta-analysis of individual patient data. *Annals of Internal Medicine* 2001;**134**:370–9.

234. Kvetny J, Gregersen G, Pedersen RS. Randomized placebo-controlled trial of perindopril in normotensive, normoalbuminuric patients with type 1 diabetes mellitus. *Quarterly Journal of Medicine* 2001;**94**:89–94.

235. Jerums G, Allen TJ, Campbell DJ *et al.* Long-term comparison between perindopril and nifedipine in normotensive patients with type 1 diabetes and microalbuminuria. *American Journal of Kidney Diseases* 2001;**37**:890–9.

236. Tarnow L, Rossing P, Jensen C *et al.* Long-term renoprotective effect of nisoldipine and lisinopril in type 1 diabetic patients with diabetic nephropathy. *Diabetes Care* 2000;**23**:1725–30.

237. Kopf D, Schmitz H, Beyer J *et al.* A double-blind trial of perindopril and nitrendipine in incipient diabetic nephropathy. *Diabetes, Nutrition and Metabolism – Clinical and Experimental* 2001;**14**:245–52.

238. Waugh NR, Robertson AM. Protein restriction for diabetic renal disease. Cochrane Database of Systematic Reviews 2002; Issue 2, 2002.

239. Zarazaga A, Lopez-Martinez, Lorenzo V *et al.* Nutritional support in chronic renal failure: systematic review. *Clinical Nutrition* 2001;**20**:291–9.

240. Hansen HP, Tauber-Lassen E, Jensen BR, Parving HH. Effect of dietary protein restriction on prognosis in patients with diabetic nephropathy. *Kidney International* 2002;**62**:220–8.

241. Meloni C, Morosetti M, Suraci C *et al.* Severe dietary protein restriction in overt diabetic nephropathy: benefits or risks? *Journal of Renal Nutrition* 2002;**12**:96–101.

242. Rossing P, Hansen BV, Nielsen FS *et al.* Fish oil in diabetic nephropathy. *Diabetes Care* 1996;**19**:1214–9.

243. National Institute for Clinical Excellence. *Management of Type 2 diabetes: renal disease – prevention and early management.* London: NICE, 2002.

244. National Institute for Clinical Excellence. *Clinical guidelines for Type 2 diabetes: prevention and management of foot problems.* London: NICE, 2003:1–164.

245. O'Meara S, Cullum N, Majid M, Sheldon T. Systematic reviews of wound care management: (3) antimicrobial agents for chronic wounds; (4) diabetic foot ulceration. *Health Technology Assessment* 2000;**4**:1–237.

246. Mayfield JA, Sugarman JR. The use of the Semmes-Weinstein monofilament and other threshold tests for preventing foot ulceration and amputation in persons with diabetes. Review. *Journal of Family Practice* 2000;**49**(11 Suppl):S17–29.

247. Paisley AN, Abbott CA, Van Schie CH, Boulton AJ. A comparison of the Neuropen against standard quantitative sensory-threshold measures for assessing peripheral nerve function. *Diabetic Medicine* 2002;**19**:400–5.

248. Bowering CK. Diabetic foot ulcers. Pathophysiology, assessment, and therapy. *Canadian Family Physician* 2001;**47**:1007–16.

249. Ackerman MD, D'Attilio JP, Antoni MH, Campbell BM. Assessment of erectile dysfunction in diabetic men: the clinical relevance of self-reported sexual functioning. *Journal of Sex and Marital Therapy* 1991;**17**:191–202.

250. Wellmer A, Sharief MK, Knowles CH *et al.* Quantitative sensory and autonomic testing in male diabetic patients with erectile dysfunction. *British Journal of Urology International* 1999;**83**:66–70.

251. Leedom L, Feldman M, Procci W, Zeidler A. Symptoms of sexual dysfunction and depression in diabetic women. *Journal of Diabetic Complications* 1991;**5**:38–41.

252. Benbow SJ, Chan AW, Bowsher DR *et al.* The prediction of diabetic neuropathic plantar foot ulceration by liquid-crystal contact thermography. *Diabetes Care* 1994;**17**:835–9.

253. Price DE, Gingell JC, Gepi-Attee S *et al.* Sildenafil: study of a novel oral treatment for erectile dysfunction in diabetic men. *Diabetic Medicine* 1998;**15**:821–5.

254. Levitt NS, Stansberry KB, Wynchank S, Vinik AI. The natural progression of autonomic neuropathy and autonomic function tests in a cohort of people with IDDM. *Diabetes Care* 1996;**19**:751–4.

255. Ryder RE, Dent MT, Ward JD. Testing for diabetic neuropathy, part two: autonomic neuropathy. *Practical Diabetes* 1992;**9**:56–60.

256. Ewing DJ, Clarke BF. Autonomic neuropathy: its diagnosis and prognosis. Review. *Clinical Endocrinology and Metabolism* 1986;**15**:855–88.

257. Gill JS, Williams G, Ghatei MA *et al.* Effect of the aldose reductase inhibitor, ponalrestat, on diabetic neuropathy. *Diabète et Métabolisme* 1990;**16**:296–302.

258. Faes TJ, Yff GA, DeWeerdt O *et al.* Treatment of diabetic autonomic neuropathy with an aldose reductase inhibitor. *Journal of Neurology* 1993;**240**:156–60.

259. Sundkvist G, Armstrong FM, Bradbury JE *et al.* Peripheral and autonomic nerve function in 259 diabetic patients with peripheral neuropathy treated with ponalrestat (an aldose reductase inhibitor) or placebo for 18 months. *Journal of Diabetes and its Complications* 1992;**6**:123–30.

260. Didangelos TP, Karamitsos DT, Athyros VG, Kourtoglou GI. Effect of aldose reductase inhibition on cardiovascular reflex tests in patients with definite diabetic autonomic neuropathy over a period of 2 years. *Journal of Diabetes and its Complications* 1998;**12**:201–7.

261. Kontopoulos AG, Athyros VG, Didangelos TP *et al.* Effect of chronic quinapril administration on heart rate variability in patients with diabetic autonomic neuropathy. *Diabetes Care* 1997;**20**:355–61.

262. Athyros VG, Didangelos TP, Karamitsos DT *et al.* Long-term effect of converting enzyme inhibition on circadian sympathetic and parasympathetic modulation in patients with diabetic autonomic neuropathy. *Acta Cardiologica* 1998;**53**:201–9.

263. Wehrmann T, Lembcke B, Caspary WF. Influence of cisapride on antroduodenal motor function in healthy subjects and diabetics with autonomic neuropathy. *Alimentary Pharmacology and Therapeutics* 1991;**5**:599–608.

264. Desautels SG, Hutson WR, Christian PE *et al.* Gastric emptying response to variable oral erythromycin dosing in diabetic gastroparesis. *Digestive Diseases and Sciences* 1995;**40**:141–6.

265. Samsom M, Jebbink RJ, Akkermans LM *et al.* Effects of oral erythromycin on fasting and postprandial antroduodenal motility in patients with type I diabetes, measured with an ambulatory manometric technique. *Diabetes Care* 1997;**20**:129–34.

266. Janssens J, Peeters TL, Vantrappen G *et al.* Improvement of gastric emptying in diabetic gastroparesis by erythromycin. Preliminary studies. *New England Journal of Medicine* 1990;**322**:1028–31.

267. Collins SL, Moore RA, McQuay HJ, Wiffen P. Antidepressants and anticonvulsants for diabetic neuropathy and postherpetic neuralgia: a quantitative systematic review. *Journal of Pain and Symptom Management* 2000;**20**:449–58.

268. Gorson KC, Schott C, Herman R *et al.* Gabapentin in the treatment of painful diabetic neuropathy: a placebo controlled, double blind, crossover trial. *Journal of Neurology, Neurosurgery and Psychiatry* 1999;**66**:251–2.

269. Eisenberg E, Lurie Y, Braker C *et al.* Lamotrigine reduces painful diabetic neuropathy: a randomized, controlled study. *Neurology* 2001;**57**:505–9.

270. Max MB, Kishore-Kumar R, Schafer SC *et al.* Efficacy of desipramine in painful diabetic neuropathy: a placebo-controlled trial. *Pain* 1991;**45**:3–9.

271. Amin P, Sturrock ND. A pilot study of the beneficial effects of amantadine in the treatment of painful diabetic peripheral neuropathy. *Diabetic Medicine* 2003;**20**:114–8.

272. Zhang WY, Po AL The effectiveness of topically applied capsaicin. A meta-analysis. *European Journal of Clinical Pharmacology* 1994;**46**:517–22.

273. Zeigler D, Lynch SA, Muir J *et al.* Transdermal clonidine versus placebo in painful diabetic neuropathy. *Pain* 1992;**48**:403–8.

274. Byas-Smith MG, Max MB, Muir J, Kingman A. Transdermal clonidine compared to placebo in painful diabetic neuropathy using a two-stage 'enriched enrollment' design. *Pain* 1995;**60**:267–74.

275. Jamal GA, Carmichael H. The effect of gamma-linolenic acid on human diabetic peripheral neuropathy: a double-blind placebo-controlled trial. *Diabetic Medicine* 1990;**7**:319–23.

276. Keen H, Payan J, Allawi J *et al.* Treatment of diabetic neuropathy with gamma-linolenic acid. The gamma-Linolenic Acid Multicenter Trial Group. *Diabetes Care* 1993;**16**:8–15.

277. Yuen KC, Baker NR, Rayman G. Treatment of chronic painful diabetic neuropathy with isosorbide dinitrate spray: a double-blind placebo-controlled cross-over study. *Diabetes Care* 2002;**25**:1699–703.

278. Oskarsson P, Ljunggren JG, Lins PE. Efficacy and safety of mexiletine in the treatment of painful diabetic neuropathy. The Mexiletine Study Group. *Diabetes Care* 1997;**20**:1594–7.

279. Stracke H, Meyer UE, Schumacher HE, Federlin K. Mexiletine in the treatment of diabetic neuropathy. *Diabetes Care* 1992;**15**:1550–5.

280. Morello CM, Leckband SG, Stoner CP *et al.* Randomized double-blind study comparing the efficacy of gabapentin with amitriptyline on diabetic peripheral neuropathy pain. *Archives of Internal Medicine* 1999;**159**:1931–7.

281. Harati Y, Gooch C, Swenson M *et al.* Double-blind randomized trial of tramadol for the treatment of the pain of diabetic neuropathy. *Neurology* 1998;**50**:1842–6.

282. Diabetes UK. *Recommendations for the management of diabetes in primary care.* London: Diabetes UK, 2000. http://www.diabetes.org.uk/infocentre/index.html

283. Department of Veterans Affairs. *The management of diabetes mellitus in the primary care setting.* US Department of Defense, 1999.

284. *Inpatient management guidelines for people with diabetes.* Nashville, TN: American Healthways, 2002.

285. Standards of medical care for patients with diabetes mellitus. *Diabetes Care* 2003;**26**:S33–50.

286. Piters KM, Kumar D, Pei E, Bessman AN. Comparison of continuous and intermittent intravenous insulin therapies for diabetic ketoacidosis. *Diabetologia* 1977;**13**:317–21.

287. Sacks HS, Shahshahani M, Kitabchi AE *et al.* Similar responsiveness of diabetic ketoacidosis to low-dose insulin by intramuscular injection and albumin-free infusion. *Annals of Internal Medicine* 1979;**90**:36–42.

288. Fisher JN, Shahshahani MN, Kitabchi AE. Diabetic ketoacidosis: low-dose insulin therapy by various routes. *New England Journal of Medicine* 1977;**297**:238–41.

289. Storms FE, Lutterman JA, van't Laar A. Comparison of efficacy of human and porcine insulin in treatment of diabetic ketoacidosis. *Diabetes Care* 1987;**10**:49–55.

290. Wiggam MI, O'Kane MJ, Harper R *et al.* Treatment of diabetic ketoacidosis using normalization of blood 3-hydroxybutyrate concentration as the endpoint of emergency management. A randomized controlled study. *Diabetes Care* 1997;**20**:1347–52.

291. Gamba G, Oseguera J, Castrejon M, Gomez-Perez FJ. Bicarbonate therapy in severe diabetic ketoacidosis. A double blind, randomized, placebo controlled trial. *Revista de Investigacion Clinica* 1991;**43**:234–8.

292. Morris LR, Murphy MB, Kitabchi AE. Bicarbonate therapy in severe diabetic ketoacidosis. *Annals of Internal Medicine* 1986;**105**:836–40.

293. Viallon A, Zeni F, Lafond P *et al.* Does bicarbonate therapy improve the management of severe diabetic ketoacidosis? *Critical Care Medicine* 1999;**27**:2690–3.

294. Fisher JN, Kitabchi AE. A randomized study of phosphate therapy in the treatment of diabetic ketoacidosis. *Journal of Clinical Endocrinology and Metabolism* 1983;**57**:177–80.

295. Wilson HK, Keuer SP, Lea AS *et al.* Phosphate therapy in diabetic ketoacidosis. *Archives of Internal Medicine* 1982;**142**:517–20.

296. Yun YS, Lee HC, Park CS *et al.* Effects of long-acting somatostatin analogue (Sandostatin) on manifest diabetic ketoacidosis. *Journal of Diabetes and its Complications* 1999;**13**:288–92.

297. Davies M, Dixon S, Currie CJ *et al.* Evaluation of a hospital diabetes specialist nursing service: a randomized controlled trial. *Diabetic Medicine* 2001;**18**:301–7.

298. Cavan DA, Hamilton P, Everett J, Kerr D. Reducing hospital inpatient length of stay for patients with diabetes. *Diabetic Medicine* 2001;**18**:162–4.

299. Rassias AJ, Marrin CA, Arruda J *et al.* Insulin infusion improves neutrophil function in diabetic cardiac surgery patients. *Anesthesia and Analgesia* 1999;**88**:1011–6.

300. Furnary AP, Zerr KJ, Grunkemeier GL, Starr A. Continuous intravenous insulin infusion reduces the incidence of deep sternal wound infection in diabetic patients after cardiac surgical procedures. *Annals of Thoracic Surgery* 1999;**67**:352–60.

301. Raucoules-Aime M, Lugrin D, Boussofara M *et al.* Intraoperative glycaemic control in non-insulin-dependent and insulin-dependent diabetes. *British Journal of Anaesthesia* 1994;**73**:443–9.

302. Christiansen CL, Schurizek BA, Malling B *et al.* Insulin treatment of the insulin-dependent diabetic patient undergoing minor surgery. Continuous intravenous infusion compared with subcutaneous administration. *Anaesthesia* 1988;**43**:533–7.

303. Pezzarossa A, Taddei F, Cimicchi MC *et al.* Perioperative management of diabetic subjects. Subcutaneous versus intravenous insulin administration during glucose-potassium infusion. *Diabetes Care* 1988;**11**:52–8.

304. Simmons D, Morton K, Laughton SJ, Scott DJ. A comparison of two intravenous insulin regimens among surgical patients with insulin-dependent diabetes mellitus. *Diabetes Educator* 1994;**20**:422–7.

305. Dazzi D, Taddei F, Gavarini A *et al.* The control of blood glucose in the critical diabetic patient: a neuro-fuzzy method. *Journal of Diabetes and its Complications* 2001;**15**:80–7.

306. Malmberg K, Ryden L, Efendic S *et al.* Randomized trial of insulin-glucose infusion followed by subcutaneous insulin treatment in diabetic patients with acute myocardial infarction (DIGAMI study): effects on mortality at 1 year. *Journal of the American College of Cardiology* 1995;**26**:57–65.

307. Malmberg KA, Efendic S, Ryden LE. Feasibility of insulin-glucose infusion in diabetic patients with acute myocardial infarction. A report from the multicenter trial: DIGAMI. *Diabetes Care* 1994;**17**:1007–14.

308. Clark RS, English M, McNeill GP, Newton RW. Effect of intravenous infusion of insulin in diabetics with acute myocardial infarction. *British Medical Journal* 1985;**291**:303–5.

309. Davis RE, McCann VJ, Stanton KG. Type 1 diabetes and latent pernicious anaemia. *Medical Journal of Australia* 1992;**156**:160–2.

310. Talal AH, Murray JA, Goeken JA, Sivitz WI. Celiac disease in an adult population with insulin-dependent diabetes mellitus: use of endomysial antibody testing. *American Journal of Gastroenterology* 1997;**92**: 1280–4.

311. Sjoberg K, Eriksson KF, Bredberg A *et al*. Screening for coeliac disease in adult insulin-dependent diabetes mellitus. *Journal of Internal Medicine* 1998;**243**:133–40.

312. Matteucci E, Cinapri V, Quilici S *et al*. Screening for coeliac disease in families of adults with Type 1 diabetes based on serological markers. *Diabetes, Nutrition and Metabolism – Clinical and Experimental* 2001;**14**:37–42.

313. Sategna-Guidetti C, Grosso S, Pulitano R *et al*. Celiac disease and insulin-dependent diabetes mellitus. Screening in an adult population. *Digestive Diseases and Sciences* 1994;**39**:1633–7.

314. Johnston SD, Ritchie C, Robinson J. Application of red cell distribution width to screening for coeliac disease in insulin-dependent diabetes mellitus. *Irish Journal of Medical Science* 1999;**168**:167–70.

315. Van Tilburg MA, McCaskill CC, Lane JD *et al*. Depressed mood is a factor in glycemic control in type 1 diabetes. *Psychosomatic Medicine* 2001;**63**:551–5.

316. Lustman PJ, Clouse RE, Carney RM. Depression and the reporting of diabetes symptoms. *International Journal of Psychiatry in Medicine* 1988;**18**:295–303.

317. Lustman PJ, Anderson RJ, Freedland KE *et al*. Depression and poor glycemic control: a meta-analytic review of the literature. *Diabetes Care* 2000;**23**:934–42.

318. Berlin I, Bisserbe JC, Eiber R *et al*. Phobic symptoms, particularly the fear of blood and injury, are associated with poor glycemic control in type I diabetic adults. *Diabetes Care* 1997;**20**:176–8.

319. Zambanini A, Newson RB, Maisey M, Feher MD. Injection related anxiety in insulin-treated diabetes. *Diabetes Research and Clinical Practice* 1999;**46**:239–46.

320. Anderson RJ, de Groot M, Grigsby AB *et al*. Anxiety and poor glycemic control: a meta-analytic review of the literature. *International Journal of Psychiatry in Medicine* 2002;**32**:235–47.

321. Anderson RJ, Freedland KE, Clouse RE, Lustman PJ. The prevalence of comorbid depression in adults with diabetes: a meta-analysis. *Diabetes Care* 2001;**24**:1069–78.

322. Lawrenson R, Williams J. Antidepressant use in people with diabetes. *Diabetes Primary Care* 2001;**3**:70–4.

323. Cox DJ, Gonder-Frederick L, Polonsky W *et al*. Blood glucose awareness training (BGAT-2): long-term benefits. *Diabetes Care* 2001;**24**:637–42.

324. Lustman PJ, Griffith LS, Clouse RE *et al*. Effects of nortriptyline on depression and glycemic control in diabetes: results of a double-blind, placebo-controlled trial. *Psychosomatic Medicine* 1997;**59**:241–50.

325. Lustman PJ, Freedland KE, Griffith LS, Clouse RE. Fluoxetine for depression in diabetes: a randomized double-blind placebo-controlled trial. *Diabetes Care* 2000;**23**:618–23.

326. Spiess K, Sachs G, Pietschmann P, Prager R. A program to reduce onset distress in unselected type I diabetic patients: effects on psychological variables and metabolic control. *European Journal of Endocrinology* 1995;**132**:580–6.

327. Lustman PJ, Griffith LS, Clouse RE *et al*. Effects of alprazolam on glucose regulation in diabetes. Results of double-blind, placebo-controlled trial. *Diabetes Care* 1995;**18**:1133–9.

328. Bryden KS, Neil A, Mayou RA *et al.* Eating habits, body weight, and insulin misuse. A longitudinal study of teenagers and young adults with type 1 diabetes. *Diabetes Care* 1999;**22**:1956–60.

329. Rodin G, Olmsted MP, Rydall AC *et al.* Eating disorders in young women with type 1 diabetes mellitus. *Journal of Psychosomatic Research* 2002;**53**:943–9.

330. Herpertz S, Wagener R, Albus C *et al.* Diabetes mellitus and eating disorders: a multicenter study on the comorbidity of the two diseases. *Journal of Psychosomatic Research* 1998;**44**:503–15.

331. Nielsen S. Eating disorders in females with type 1 diabetes: an update of a meta-analysis. *European Eating Disorders Review* 2002;**10**:241–54.

332. Alloway SC, Toth EL, McCargar LJ. Effectiveness of a group psychoeducation program for the treatment of subclinical disordered eating in women with type 1 diabetes. *Canadian Journal of Dietetic Practice and Research* 2001;**62**:188–92.

333. Affenito SG, Kerstetter J. Position of the American Dietetic Association and Dietitians of Canada: women's health and nutrition. *Journal of the American Dietetic Association* 1999;**99**:738–51.

334. Rose M, Hildebrandt M, Fliege H *et al.* Relevance of the treatment facility for disease-related knowledge of diabetic patients. *Diabetes Care* 2000;**23**:1708–9.

335. Diabetes Integrated Care Evaluation Team. Integrated care for diabetes: clinical, psychosocial, and economic evaluation. *British Medical Journal* 1994;**308**:1208–12.

336. Fukunishi I, Horikawa N, Yamazaki T *et al.* Perception and utilization of social support in diabetic control. *Diabetes Research and Clinical Practice* 1998;**41**:207–11.

337. Connell CM, Davis WK, Gallant MP, Sharpe PA. Impact of social support, social cognitive variables, and perceived threat on depression among adults with diabetes. *Health Psycholology* 1994;**13**:263–73.

338. Loveman E, Cave C, Green C *et al.* The clinical and cost-effectiveness of patient education models for diabetes: a systematic review and economic evaluation. *Health Technology Assessment.* 2003;**7**:iii, 1–iii190.

339. Glasgow RE, La Chance PA, Toobert DJ *et al.* Long-term effects and costs of brief behavioural dietary intervention for patients with diabetes delivered from the medical office. *Patient Education and Counseling* 1997;**32**:175–84.

340. Kaplan RM, Hartwell SL, Wilson DK, Wallace JP. Effects of diet and exercise interventions on control and quality of life in non-insulin-dependent diabetes mellitus. *Journal of General Internal Medicine* 1987;**2**:220–8.

341. Starostina EG, Antsiferov M, Galstyan GR *et al.* Effectiveness and cost-benefit analysis of intensive treatment and teaching programmes for type 1 (insulin-dependent) diabetes mellitus in Moscow – blood glucose versus urine glucose self-monitoring. *Diabetologia* 1994;**37**:170–6.

342. Dranitsaris G, Longo CJ, Grossman LD. The economic value of a new insulin preparation, Humalog Mix 25. Measured by a willingness-to-pay approach. *Pharmacoeconomics* 2000;**18**:275–87.

343. Lifetime benefits and costs of intensive therapy as practiced in the diabetes control and complications trial. The Diabetes Control and Complications Trial Research Group. *Journal of the American Medical Association* 1996;**276**:1409–15.

344. Palmer AJ, Sendi PP, Spinas GA. Applying some UK Prospective Diabetes Study results to Switzerland: the cost-effectiveness of intensive glycaemic control with metformin versus conventional control in overweight patients with type-2 diabetes. *Schweizerische medizinische Wochenschrift* 2000;**130**:1034–40.

345. Herman WH, Dasbach EJ, Songer TJ, Eastman RC. The cost-effectiveness of intensive therapy for diabetes mellitus. *Endocrinology and Metabolism Clinics of North America* 1997;**26**:679–95.

346. Stern Z, Levy R. Analysis of direct cost of standard compared with intensive insulin treatment of insulin-dependent diabetes mellitus and cost of complications. *Acta Diabetolica* 1996;**33**:48–52.

347. Graff MR,. McClanahan MA. Assessment by patients with diabetes mellitus of two insulin pen delivery systems versus a vial and syringe. *Clinical Therapeutics* 1998;**20**:486–96.

348. Hornquist JO, Wikby A, Stenstrom U, Andersson PO. Change in quality of life along with type 1 diabetes. *Diabetes Research and Clinical Practice* 1995;**28**:63–72.

349. Hornquist JO, Wikby A, Andersson PO, Dufva AM. Insulin-pen treatment, quality of life and metabolic control: retrospective intra-group evaluations. *Diabetes Research and Clinical Practice* 1990;**10**:221–30.

350. Jonsson B, Cook JR, Pedersen TR. The cost-effectiveness of lipid lowering in patients with diabetes: results from the 4S trial. *Diabetologia* 1999;**42**:1293–301.

351. Grover SA, Coupal L, Zowall H, Dorais M. Cost-effectiveness of treating hyperlipidemia in the presence of diabetes : who should be treated? *Circulation* 2000;**102**:722–7.

352. Grover SA, Coupal L, Zowall H *et al*. How cost-effective is the treatment of dyslipidemia in patients with diabetes but without cardiovascular disease? *Diabetes Care* 2001;**24**:45–50.

353. Grover SA, Levinton C, Paquet S. Identifying adults at low risk for significant hyperlipidemia: a validated clinical index. *Journal of Clinical Epidemiology* 1999;**52**:49–55.

354. Javitt JC, Canner JK, Sommer A. Cost effectiveness of current approaches to the control of retinopathy in type I diabetics. *Ophthalmology* 1989;**96**:255–64.

355. Javitt JC, Canner JK, Frank RG *et al*. Detecting and treating retinopathy in patients with type I diabetes mellitus. A health policy model. *Ophthalmology* 1990;**97**:483–94.

356. Javitt JC, Aiello LP, Bassi LJ *et al*. Detecting and treating retinopathy in patients with type I diabetes mellitus. Savings associated with improved implementation of current guidelines. American Academy of Ophthalmology. *Ophthalmology* 1991;**98**:1565–73.

357. Fendrick AM, Javitt JC, Chiang YP. Cost-effectiveness of the screening and treatment of diabetic retinopathy. What are the costs of underutilization? *International Journal of Technology Assessment in Health Care* 1992;**8**:694–707.

358. Javitt JC,.Aiello LP. Cost-effectiveness of detecting and treating diabetic retinopathy. *Annals of Internal Medicine* 1996;**124**:164–9.

359. Crijns H, Casparie AF, Hendrikse F. Continuous computer simulation analysis of the cost-effectiveness of screening and treating diabetic retinopathy. *International Journal of Technology Assessment in Health Care* 1999;**15**:198–206.

360. Polak BC, Crijns H, Casparie AF, Niessen LW. Cost-effectiveness of glycemic control and ophthalmological care in diabetic retinopathy. *Health Policy* 2003;**64**:89–97.

361. Bjorvig S, Johansen MA, Fossen K. An economic analysis of screening for diabetic retinopathy. *Journal of Telemedicine and Telecare* 2002;**8**:32–5.

362. Maberley D, Walker H, Koushik A, Cruess A. Screening for diabetic retinopathy in James Bay, Ontario: a cost-effectiveness analysis. *Canadian Medical Association Journal* 2003;**168**:160–4.

363. Pegoraro A, Singh A, Bakir AA, Arruda JA, Dunea G. Simplified screening for microalbuminuria. *Annals of Internal Medicine* 1997;**127**:817–9.

364. Lewis JB. Microalbuminuria: accuracy or economics. *American Journal of Kidney Diseases* 1998;**32**:524–8.

365. Faronato P, de Bigontina G. A cost-benefit analysis of two mass screening strategies for albuminuria in diabetic patients. *Diabetes, Nutrition & Metabolism: Clinical and Experimental* 1994;7(6):325–329.

366. Le Floch JP. Cost effectiveness of screening for microalbuminuria. *Diabetic Medicine* 1994;**11**:349–356: (Abstract)

367. Hendry BM, Viberti GC, Hummel S *et al*. Modelling and costing the consequences of using an ACE inhibitor to slow the progression of renal failure in type I diabetic patients. *Quarterly Journal of Medicine* 1997;**90**:277–82.

368. Garattini L, Brunetti M, Salvioni F, Barosi M. Economic evaluation of ACE Inhibitor treatment of nephropathy in patients with insulin-dependent diabetes mellitus in Italy. *Pharmacoeconomics* 1997;**12**:67–75.

369. Rodby RA, Firth LM, Lewis EJ. An economic analysis of captopril in the treatment of diabetic nephropathy. The Collaborative Study Group. *Diabetes Care* 1996;**19**:1051–61.

370. Clark WF, Churchill DN, Forwell L *et al.* To pay or not to pay? A decision and cost-utility analysis of angiotensin-converting-enzyme inhibitor therapy for diabetic nephropathy. *Canadian Medical Association Journal* 2000;**162**:195–8.

371. van Os N, Niessen LW, Bilo HJ *et al.* Diabetes nephropathy in the Netherlands: a cost effectiveness analysis of national clinical guidelines. *Health Policy* 2000;**51**:135–47.

372. Borch-Johnsen K, Wenzel H, Viberti GC, Mogensen CE. Is screening and intervention for microalbuminuria worthwhile in patients with insulin dependent diabetes? *British Medical Journal* 1993;**306**:1722–5.

373. Kiberd BA, Jindal KK. Screening to prevent renal failure in insulin dependent diabetic patients: an economic evaluation. *British Medical Journal* 1995;**311**:1595–9.

374. Siegel JE, Krolewski AS, Warram JH, Weinstein MC. Cost-effectiveness of screening and early treatment of nephropathy in patients with insulin-dependent diabetes mellitus. *Journal of the American Society of Nephrology* 1992;**3**:S111–S119.

375. Palmer AJ, Weiss C, Sendi PP, Neeser K, Brandt A, Singh G *et al.* The cost-effectiveness of different management strategies for type I diabetes: a Swiss perspective. *Diabetologia* 2000;**43**:13–26.

376. Allenet B, Paree F, Lebrun T, Carr L, Posnett J, Martini J *et al.* Cost-effectiveness modeling of Dermagraft for the treatment of diabetic foot ulcers in the French context. *Diabetes and Metabolism* 2000;**26**:125–32.

377. University of York Health Economics Consortium. *Evaluation of the cost-effectiveness of Dermagraft for the treatment of diabetic foot ulcers in the UK.* York: YHEC, 1997.

378. Kowalske KJ, Agre JC. Neuromuscular rehabilitation and electrodiagnosis. 3. Generalized peripheral neuropathy. *Archives of Physical Medicine and Rehabilitation* 2000;**81**:S20–S26.

379. Javor KA, Kotsanos JG, McDonald RC *et al.* Diabetic ketoacidosis charges relative to medical charges of adult patients with type I diabetes. *Diabetes Care* 1997;**20**:349–54.

380. Davey P, Grainger D, MacMillan J *et al.* Economic evaluation of insulin lispro versus neutral (regular) insulin therapy using a willingness-to-pay approach. *Pharmacoeconomics* 1998;**13**:347–58.

381. Wu SY, Lung BC, Chang S *et al.* Evaluation of drug usage and expenditure in a hospital diabetes clinic. *Journal of Clinical Pharmacy and Therapeutics* 1998;**23**:49–56.

382. McIntosh A, Hutchinson A, Home PD *et al.* *Clinical guidelines and evidence review for Type 2 diabetes: management of blood glucose.* Sheffield: ScHARR, University of Sheffield, 2001.